REIKI

Energy healing Guide To Learning reiki symbols and acquiring tips for reiki meditation

(Learn Reiki healing and improve health and reduce stress)

William Campion

Published by Rob Miles

William Campion

All Rights Reserved

Reiki: Energy healing Guide To Learning reiki symbols and acquiring tips for reiki meditation (Learn Reiki healing and improve health and reduce stress)

ISBN 978-1-989990-24-7

All rights reserved. No part of this guide may be reproduced in any form without permission in writing from the publisher except in the case of brief quotations embodied in critical articles or reviews.

Legal & Disclaimer

The information contained in this book is not designed to replace or take the place of any form of medicine or professional medical advice. The information in this book has been provided for educational and entertainment purposes only.

The information contained in this book has been compiled from sources deemed reliable, and it is accurate to the best of the Author's knowledge; however, the Author cannot guarantee its accuracy and validity and cannot be held liable for any errors or omissions. Changes are periodically made to this book. You must consult your doctor or get professional medical advice before using any of the suggested remedies, techniques, or information in this book.

Upon using the information contained in this book, you agree to hold harmless the Author from and against any damages, costs, and expenses, including any legal fees potentially resulting from the application of any of the information provided by this guide. This disclaimer applies to any damages or injury caused by the use and application, whether directly or indirectly, of any advice or information presented, whether for breach of contract, tort, negligence, personal injury, criminal intent, or under any other cause of action.

You agree to accept all risks of using the information presented inside this book. You need to consult a professional medical practitioner in order to ensure you are both able and healthy enough to participate in this program.

Table of Contents

INTRODUCTION 1

CHAPTER 1: JUST WHAT IS REIKI? 8

CHAPTER 2: ETHICS OF ENERGY WORK 12

CHAPTER 3: HOW CAN REIKI HEALING HELP ME? 19

CHAPTER 4: ABOUT REIKI 21

CHAPTER 5: HOW DOES REIKI HEAL? 35

CHAPTER 6: HAND PLACEMENT FOR HEALING YOURSELF 52

CHAPTER 7: CREATING A HEALING PARTNERSHIP. 67

CHAPTER 8: MEDITATION TECHNIQUES TO HARNESS THE POWER OF REIKI 75

CHAPTER 9: SYMBOLS 83

CHAPTER 10: THE INTRICACIES OF INTENTION SETTING .. 91

CHAPTER 11: DEVELOPING YOUR REIKI PRACTICE 101

CHAPTER 12: WESTERN / TRADITIONAL REIKI - DIFFERENCE? 112

CHAPTER 13: THE IMPORTANCE OF INITIATION SIZE 116

CHAPTER 14: BENEFITS OF HEALING ENERGY 138

CHAPTER 15: REIKI ATTUNEMENT 146

CHAPTER 16: SYMBOLS IN REIKI 152

CHAPTER 17: WHO CAN PRACTICE REIKI 158

CHAPTER 18: MASSIVE SYNCHRONICITY 175

CONCLUSION 188

Introduction

Reiki is taken into consideration an organic approach of recovery by producing as well as promoting the global life pressure we have. The specialist either areas their hands gently on or over different locations of the person's physical body to promote the transfer of Ki. Throughout the therapy, the individuals possess recovery reactions are meant to be promoted.

Reiki which is certainly a kind of power recovery entails the straight application of Ki (Chinese spell it Qi) for the objective of enhancing the customers power area or mood. Both Scientific research and also individuals that are spiritual both think that the hidden factor for the recovery is believed as the type of power excitement. An instance would certainly be an individual that is unwell and also prays as well as instantly the health problem starts to decrease.

When one undertakes a Reiki therapy, the Reiki professional makes use of Ki to re straighten the individual obtaining the Reiki therapy's biography area recognized as a mood and also their physical body right into an unified state. It is thought that via the customer's loosened up state that the mind and also physical body straighten themselves via the support of the instructions of Ki via the expert's hands.

Reiki is thought about a holistic medicine and also a spiritual recovery type. It uses resonances that are moved from the professional to the individual obtaining the therapy using the specialist's hands. This is to produce homeostasis equilibrium and also a total feeling of wellness in the individual getting the Reiki.

The Reiki specialist songs right into this power by utilizing particular signs to call on the power for recovery functions. Reiki therapists vary from Chinese recovery like acupuncture since they do not try to unblock the Ki like Chinese Conventional Medication aims to. The Reiki Master does this by calling on the Universal power to raise their very own Ki and also after that move it to the individual obtaining the Reiki therapy.

Due to the fact that of this Reiki professionals likewise think that points that are psychological as well as spiritual could likewise be recovered as well as the physical considering that the power steps and also adjustments. Reiki heals by bring back the physical type as very closely to the concept type of our own selves that we could obtain.

Reiki specialists really feel if the vital force or Ki is reduced after that an individual could really feel anxiety, stress as well as health problem both emotionally as well as literally. If the Ki moves extremely as well as openly in our physical bodies after that it advertises maximum wellness, joy as well as health.

To be a Reiki Master one needs to find out different phases of exactly what is called Attunement. The Reiki Specialist needs to recognize just what signs to make use of, when to call the Universal Life pressure, the best ways to separate in between a psychological or spiritual ailment as well as ways to recover an individual that is not literally existing. Reiki is just one of one of the most commonly made use of power recovery techniques worldwide today.

Reiki refers to the power utilized in this recovery technique as resisted to the real strategies educated by the masters. In comparison to points like western medication where the signs are healed; Reiki establishes out to "heal" the individual's state of being to impact a modification for the far better. Reiki runs on the degree of the solidification of a power kind.

Reiki is a spiritual method established in 1922 by a Japanese Buddhist Monk by the name of Mikao Usui. The technique utilizes the hands to move the Ki of the Reiki professional to the one getting the Reiki.

In this instance an individual might look for out a Reiki master in order to attempt as well as influence a modification to recover the reason of the discomfort. Discomfort like any kind of various other psychological, behavior, physical, mental or spiritual restriction like illness is due to the fact that the individual is not straightened with their physical selves and also their excellent selves.

With Reiki, the suggestion is to locate the restriction that is stopping the individual from being a "entire" being as well as to discover as well as acknowledge the pattern then launch it right into the recovery universe so the individual could be re straightened right into a state of health and wellness. This might or might not take place on the mindful degree however the Reiki Master launches the "unwell" in a manner of speaking, so the individual could be healthy and balanced literally, mentally and also mentally.

The technique makes use of the hands to move the Ki of the Reiki specialist to the one getting the Reiki. When one goes through a Reiki therapy, the Reiki specialist makes use of Ki to re straighten the individual getting the Reiki therapy's biography area recognized as a mood and also their physical body right into an unified state. The Reiki Master does this by calling on the Universal power to raise their very own Ki and also after that move it to the individual getting the Reiki therapy. The Reiki Expert has to understand just what signs to utilize, when to call the Universal Life pressure, exactly how to separate in between a psychological or spiritual ailment and also just how to recover an individual that is not literally existing. In comparison to points like western medication where the signs and symptoms are treated; Reiki establishes out to "treat" the individual's state of being to influence a modification for the far better.

Chapter 1: Just What Is Reiki?

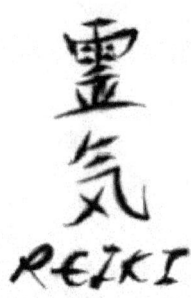

Reiki, pronounced ray-key, is a form of energy healing that manipulates the energy that flows through your body naturally. Your entire body at its core is made up of vibrating energy. You may be entirely skeptical that such a thing as this 'spiritual life force energy' could even exist. Whether it exists or not, something exists within your body to cause an electrical force that allows synapses to fire within your brain, pain signals to pass from your brain to your muscles, then back again. In addition to this, some kind of electrical communication is happening between muscles without even going to the brain!

Doctors know there is energy inside the body

Doctors use electroencephalographs (EEGs) to check the energy used by your brain, electrocardiograms (ECGs) to be sure your heart is working right and electromyography (EMGs) to see if your muscles are communicating with your nerves correctly and how fast those messages are passing.

Why can't there be some kind of life force flowing through your body that can be manipulated by someone practicing this type of energy healing?

Now, you might be thinking that Reiki is some kind of religious cult since I've mentioned it being a 'spiritual life force', but it really isn't. You don't have to believe in anything other than what you really want to believe.

Reiki is used by many cultures

Reiki is practiced by people of all types of religion, as well as those with no religious beliefs. If there is anything 'religious' about Reiki, it is that you must believe it will work for you!

Some may not believe that just waving your hands over your body can alter the natural energy flow, but it is quite true and possible. Some practitioners can do this, but many modern Reiki therapists use actual massage to help to restore the natural flow of that energy within your body. You can learn how to do that too! I know that if I hurt somewhere, the pain will just keep roiling up that energy just like big rocks in the middle of a river creates a series of rapids.

Imagine you're in a raft on a nice placid river, just floating along. You hear a low rumbling just at the edge of your hearing and when you travel around the bend in the river, there ahead of you is a set of rapids. Some rapids just make your raft bounce around a little but others can make your raft bounce, dip and spin around because the flow of the water is so disrupted by the rocks beneath the surface. Muscle pain causes these same disturbances in that energy flowing through your body, so the Reiki therapist will sometimes use regular massage techniques to ease the pain. They can then encourage that life force to flow more smoothly to take healing to the part of the body that needs it.

Reiki is not difficult to understand and it is quite easy to perform. Reiki is the use of the life force energy that occurs naturally in your body to heal your body through the belief that it will work and that the manipulation of your life force energy will facilitate that healing.

Read on to find out just how Reiki works.

Chapter 2: Ethics Of Energy Work

Shamanic Reiki is considered an energy modality and as such it comes with ethical standards which allow the practitioner to remain professional in the eyes of their clients and peers.

First and foremost, you should obtain your clients permission before working on them. Even though Reiki works for the highest good, there are several reasons why someone may not want to have energy work performed on them. The best way to earn your clients trust is to ensure you have explained what Shamanic Reiki is, how the treatment is performed, and what to expect during and after the treatment. Of course you must respect whatever decision your client makes. You may use a client consent form describing the above information and obtain a signature from your client consenting to treatment. This protects both you and your client from misunderstandings and communication errors. In the event that the client is unable to communicate, such as being comatose or is someone you don't even know, there is still a way to work with these clients. In these cases you can send Reiki with the clear intent for the persons Higher Self to determine whether or not to accept this energy. In this way you are not forcing Reiki on anyone, just ensuring that it is working towards the highest good for those involved. This is especially beneficial if you send Reiki with the request that any unused energy returns to the Earth for healing. In level 2 we will discuss the use of distance healing and treating people that are unable to be present.

While using energy work or any complementary/alternative medicine techniques, we always strongly recommend that the person seek the advice of a licensed Health Care Professional in facilitating their own wellness.

As of the publishing of this manual, there are no specific requirements for energy work in the state of North Carolina, however you must check with your individual state laws as they vary from state to state. You do not have to be licensed in any other health care modality to be a Reiki Practitioner, so Reiki is open to the public. There are stipulations to ensure that you are not practicing outside your scope of practice. As a Reiki Practitioner you may not perform any soft tissue manipulations, prescribe any remedies whether herbal or synthetic, or engage in any other activities outside the scope of a Reiki Practitioner. You may however obtain your certificate as an ordained minister to use the "laying on of hands" for energy work practice. It is recommended at the very least, to obtain this credential before beginning an energy work business.

The scope of practice for the Shamanic Reiki Practitioner includes; the consent for client treatment, assess energy field & chakras of the client, applying light touch without tissue manipulation, clear and move energy as needed for proper function, ensure the comfort of the client, maintain appropriate therapeutic relationship and always work for the highest good.

While performing Reiki treatments it is customary to apply a light touch or hover just above the clients' skin. Clients may stay clothed, or depending upon what other modalities you may provide, you may have clients draped appropriately on a treatment table. It is important to stay within your scope of practice to ensure the safety of your clients and yourself.

To further enhance your client's trust, it is important to uphold confidentiality. Any information given to you through the use of forms or conversations may not be shared. Ethics are an important part of maintaining a practitioner-client relationship. The stronger you adhere to the ethical standards, the fewer problems you will encounter as a professional. Ethical standards state that you as the practitioner should not abuse your power over the client, shall maintain appropriate records, conduct your sessions professionally, and adhere to a strict confidentiality policy. While there is no governing licensing agency to supervise our work, I do require all students to sign a contract promising to adhere to the scope of practice and ethical standards taught in this tradition upon certification.

As you do more healing work, you will begin to learn to sense problems. You have a responsibility to share this; however, it is important to be gentle in how you share this information and remember you cannot diagnose anything, but merely suggest a follow up doctor visit concerning a particular area that should be checked.

Above all else remember to do no harm. Your intent should always remain for the highest good of all people involved. Always stay within your scope of practice and maintain your professional ethical standards at all times.

While Reiki may be used for anyone, in most situations, we must be sure to keep an open mind and an open heart. There are times during treatments when symptoms are relieved immediately and of course there are times when it doesn't relieve any symptoms at all. It may take several sessions over a period of time, or may take one. Everybody is different and every situation is different. A person who is open to healing will still receive only what their highest good will allow. A person who is not open to healing will often times become less rigid and more open through Reiki. While most Reiki Practitioners have seen profound results from treatments, there are times when it seems the Reiki is not working. It is during these times that our faith in the Reiki energy is tested and we must remember to keep our hearts open and accept the outcome which may be serving the greater good in a way we cannot see and do not understand. We must trust that the energy is doing what is right for that person at that time. Reiki can be used alone with great results, or it may be combined with other modalities as well. Shamanic Reiki Therapy will not conflict with other treatments, whether conventional or complimentary. If a person is using medication, acupuncture, or herbal remedies, then Reiki will serve to harmonize those treatments as well as providing its own benefit.

Chapter 3: How Can Reiki Healing Help Me?

Individuals use Reiki to relax and enhance well-being. They reduce discomfort, depression and exhaustion. Aid in the treatment of symptoms. Remove side effects of drugs. According to a 2007 national survey, 1.2 million adults and 161,000 children have received one or more energy treatment sessions in the previous year, such as Reiki.

Reiki is a great integrative therapy to try because Reiki usually makes people feel better. Because depression and pain decrease and people expect to improve their wellbeing, they feel better able to include other needed medical treatments or to make necessary improvements to the lifestyle. Reiki therapy also clears the mind and allows patients to better assess the sometimes contradictory medical information that multiple clinicians have, allowing them to make more informed critical treatment decisions. Reiki can thus help people become more active in their own health.

Reiki can be done by someone else (either a friend, a healthcare professional or Reiki professionals), or studied by everyone who wants to practice Reiki on their own.

Reiki is currently widely used by three groups:

1.The lay public at home, family and friends

2.Professionals from Reiki offer treatment in their offices or other health and wellness facilities

3.Nurses and medical practitioners, doctors, and other health professionals including physical therapists, dentists, massage therapists, and chiropractors who integrate Reiki into healthcare during work visits or stationary care in clinics, hospitals, nursing homes, hospices and other health care centers.

Chapter 4: About Reiki

This chapter is designed to teach you everything you need to know about Reiki itself.

The History of Reiki

The English word Reiki comes from the Japanese word meaning "mysterious atmosphere" or "supernatural influence" in Chinese. Its earliest recorded usage, in English, dates back to 1975.[1,2] Instead of calling it the above names, the English language ended up translating Reiki, to meaning "universal life energy".[3]

The system of Reiki was developed by Mikao Usui in 1922 while performing a twenty-one day Buddhist training course held on Mount Kurama; likely involving: meditation, fasting, and prayer. Usui was attuned to Reiki from the universe through his crown chakra, which allowed him to practice Reiki and also attune others. In April 1922, Usui moved to Tokyo and founded the Usui Reiki Ryōhō Gakkaiso he could continue treating people on a large scale with Reiki.[2]

Usui taught his system of Reiki to over 2000 people during his lifetime, and sixteen of these students continued their training to reach the Master/Teacher degree. While teaching Reiki in Fukuyama, Usui suffered a stroke and died on 9 March 1926.[2] Reiki was then brought over to the United States, starting in Hawaii in 1938 by Takata of which was then practiced throughout the United States. Takata died December 11, 1980 of which she trained 22 Reiki Masters and almost all Reiki taught outside of Japan.[2]

The Meaning of Reiki

Reiki can be broken down to: rei meaning spirit or divine[4] and ki meaning: chi.[5]

The Reiki Principals or 5 admonitions:

1. Don't get angry today.

2. Don't be grievous.

3. Express your thanks.

4. Be diligent in your business.

5. Be kind to others.

The different types of Reiki[6]:

Usui Reiki:

Mikao Usui was the founder of reiki, which is practiced all over the world. Hawayo Takata, a Japanese woman, spread the teachings of Reiki, to the West.[6]

Tibetan Reiki:
This form of reiki is a powerful Tibetan method of attunement and combines certain techniques from the original Usui reiki. [6]

Karuna Reiki:
Karuna means a profound feeling to alleviate suffering, with abiding compassion towards all beings. Karuna Reiki employs sounds, endowed with the power to heal. These sounds are sacred

and powerful. They can be transmitted silently through intention or chanting, to bring about deeper levels of healing. The power of Karuna Reiki is used to heal addictions.

Gendai Reiki:
Gendai means modern. Mr. Hiroshi Doi is the founder of this reiki. He brings a strong Buddhist perspective to the original reiki teachings.

Rainbow Reiki:
Walter Lubeck, a reiki master began this form of reiki. In this system, working with the seven main chakras in the body brings about healing. These chakras organize a body of light. This spiritual energy is used to heal and understand our true nature.

Five Element Seichem:
Alex Baisley in Canada founded this system. This helps us to consciously use the five elements of the universal life force or prana to promote healing.

Shamballa Reiki:
This system helps to cleanse, repair and

balance the physical, emotional, mental and spiritual levels of a person. It uses reiki energy along with many vibratory symbols and healing rays to achieve the purpose. [6]

Kundalini Reiki: In this system, reiki energy is channeled through the lower base chakra rather than crown chakra. This kindles spirituality and even helps the practitioner get over shyness, or recover from trauma and other negative emotions. [6]

Imara Reiki: The Reiki energy is used to work on past life, repressed issues and helps in long distance healing. The practitioner is connected to ascended masters and angels. [6]

How Reiki Works

Reiki is energy from the universe. Much like how we talked about how everything in the universe runs on a vibration and everything is energy- Reiki is energy and it comes from the universe.

When you get attuned to Reiki, it opens your energy up to being a channel for Reiki. You receive Reiki and it flows through you. This means that you can channel Reiki through you, to heal yourself and others. Using energy from the universe, or Reiki, you can heal just about anything from physical, energetic/spiritual to emotional issues. I like to think of Reiki as a great addition to any treatment plan you already have going from your physician.

Reiki: as an Addition of Energy, Replacing Energy, Healing Energy.

When you receive Reiki, you receive energy from the universe. This energy, automatically knows where your body and energy, needs it most- so it will go there on its own. You receiving this energy can make you energized because you are receiving an addition of energy to the energy you already have. It can also be thought of that you are receiving positive energy, which will replace unwanted energies (like sick, unwell, negative, stagnant, energies) and promote healing. Because this energy is taking over the energy you have, you will be being filled with Reiki energy, allowing your body to heal itself naturally and replacing any unwanted energies with positive healing energy.

You never have to worry about whether or not you are sending too much or not enough energy. Because Reiki, not only goes where it is needed, but it knows how much the person, animal, plant, etc. needs.

What Can Be Helped

Reiki is a great complementary treatment to any ailment- no matter if it is physical, emotional, metal or spiritual/energetic. Reiki is great for everything- no matter how small or big the issue is, or how long you have been affected by it. Reiki knows what you need and how much you need. Think of Reiki as your added source for healing; that can be a great compliment to any treatment you are currently using from your physician- for anything from headaches to cancer, letting go of the past or healing from an emotionally taxing relationship, depression, or just clearing energy from a long day at work. Reiki can assist you with just about anything.

Reiki as a Complimentary Treatment

You will notice that I specify Reiki as a complimentary treatment a lot. This is simply because I feel like Reiki is a great assistance to what you do for yourself every day.

I will also note that Reiki is not a replacement for any treatment you are currently using as guided by your physician. If you take medications, or need treatments in any form- continue your regular treatments as guided by your physician. Reiki is not meant to replace anything you are told to do by your physician. Reiki is a great compliment to what you are already doing. Never advise someone to stop their regular treatments guided by their physicians.

A story: I heard a story from a Reiki practitioner once about a woman who was trying to force her client to stop taking Insulin for diabetes. From what I heard, the woman yelled at the client, telling him to stop using it. This situation really aggravates me, because if you are specifically told by your doctor or other health care professional, to use or do something- DO NOT stop it unless advised by that medical professional. Reiki does not replace traditional treatments for any ailment, disease, etc. and it is to be used in addition to what you are doing currently. Never tell someone to stop taking medications, or to stop treatments they are advised to do by a medical professional.

Your Body as a Channel for Reiki Energy

When you watch television the cable company sends the programming through wires that connect to your television so you can watch it. Reiki works in a similar way. Reiki energy, from the universe, flows into and down through your crown chakra and out your hands. This is why you shouldn't feel drained after providing Reiki, because you are not using your own energy, the energy is being taken in, from a higher source, flowed through you and out your hands. You can also channel Reiki to use for yourself or for distant healing, of which it doesn't need to flow out of your hands- Reiki, in an energy that flows through you from your crown chakra, and is facilitated with the use of symbols.

About Reiki Attunements and Symbols

To practice Reiki you need symbols to activate the flow of energy. You obtain the symbols during your class by being attuned to the energy with symbols. An attunement is the opening of your aura, of which the Reiki symbols are gently placed within it and then your aura is closed back up.

How to Receive Reiki and Self Healing

To receive Reiki yourself and facilitate self healing you must activate the symbol(s) you have been attuned to and then go ahead with the healing in one of two ways.

1. The first way you can facilitate a self healing is by activating the Reiki symbols and letting the Reiki energy flow through you and take over your energy. Then when you are done, you can close it back up.

2. The second way you can facilitate a self healing is by activating the Reiki symbols and then actually using your hands to heal you using different hand positions below- like you would facilitate healing for someone else.

There is more information about this in Chapter 5.

How to Give Reiki

To give Reiki to someone else or to a plant, animal, etc. You must activate the Reiki symbols and then go ahead with the healing, using both your intuition and the hand positions below. Before giving Reiki you would set an intention as preparation, and after the session, you would close the person's energy to Reiki. There will be more information about this below- in chapter 6.

The Cleansing Period

It is important to know, and also to tell clients, that sometimes they can experience a cleansing process after receiving a Reiki treatment or Reiki attunement.

A cleansing period, also called A Healing Crisis or Detoxification- is when your body releases energy that no longer serves it. Usually, this energy is unhealthy energy, negative energy, sick energy, etc. that has been released during the Reiki treatment or attunement and it was replaced with healthy energy.

The release can be experienced physically, for example, runny nose, flu-like symptoms, bowel movements, urination, etc. or through emotional release like: crying, etc.

The visualization is: Think of this- when you get a cold, the unhealthy stuff like mucus and phlegm usually comes out through your nose or through coughing. This is how your body is getting rid of that sickness from your body. It is a similar concept with the Reiki cleansing period.

Different Uses for Reiki

You can use Reiki for just about anything you wish. Reiki is not limited to treatments, healing and attunements. Reiki can be used to enhance the healing properties of water or food. You can give Reiki to anything you consume. You can use Reiki during your yoga sessions, and other movement exercises or stress reduction exercises. Reiki can help you in times of stress or even in tough situation- for example: if you are stuck in a traffic jam. By giving the situation Reiki, you will be surprised at how much easier the traffic moves and how much less stressed you are. Reiki can be given to anything and used for anything. Be creative and make Reiki work for you.

Chapter 5: How Does Reiki Heal?

We are alive because life force is flowing through us. Life force flows within the physical body through pathways called Chakras, meridian and nadis. It also flows around us in a field of energy called the Aura. Life force nourishes the organs and cells of the body, supporting them in their vital functions. When this flow of life force is disrupted /blocked, it causes diminished function in the organs and tissues of the physical body.

The life force is responsive to thoughts and feelings. It becomes disrupted when we accept, either consciously or unconsciously, negative thoughts or feelings about ourselves. These negative thoughts and feelings attach themselves to the energy field and cause a disruption in the flow of life force. This diminishes the vital function of the organs and cells of the physical body.

Reiki heals by flowing through the affected parts of the energy field and charging them with positive energy. It raises the vibratory level of the energy field in and around the physical body where the negative thoughts and feeling are attached. This causes the negative energy to break apart and fall way. In doing so, Reiki clears the energy pathways, thus allowing the life force to flow in a healthy and natural way. Therefore, Reiki balances, harmonizes and heals the physical, etheric, emotional and mental bodies. It replenishes the life force energy, clears energy blocks, increases the vitality of the body, relives stress & pain, cleanses the body of toxins, shortens the healing time of injuries and sickness, induces deep relaxation and basically increases the positive and decreases the negative in the bodies.

What can Reiki be used for?

Self-healing and healing others on all levels (physical, etheric, emotional & mental).

First-aid – giving Reiki immediately after the injured by placing the hands on the injured area helps to heal, reduce the healing time ad calm the injured person. In case of fainting, putting the hands of the soles of the feet, sending Reiki up through the body can help.

Animal – Reiki can be used to treat animals, and will have the same affects like humans.

Plants – Reiki can be used on plants to increase their growth.

Food – Reiki can be given to food in order to increase the Ki in food and clear the food from negative emotions/energies that were put into the food by the cooker.

Benefits of Reiki

Physical Benefits

Physical pain in general

Helps in digestion

Accelerates the body's self-healing ability

Migraines and headaches

Back pain

Heart disease

Asthma

Reduce pain after surgery

Prepares the body for surgery

Quickens recovery time after surgery

Reduce blood pressure

Supports the immune system

Supports pregnancy and childbirth

Assists the body in cleansing itself from toxins

Compliments medical treatment.

Mental and emotional benefits

Dissolves energy blocks and promotes natural balance between mind, body and spirit (stress, depression, anxiety, fear, worry, sadness and other unhealthy feeling)

Clears the mind and improves focus

Improves memory

Increases self-confidence

Aids better sleep

Spiritual benefits

Helps spiritual growth

Enhances meditative states

However, Reiki does not promise a miraculous cure from disease. Conditions that have taken years to manifest in the physical body cannot be cures in a few sessions. The person has to want to be well and will probably also need to make some lifestyle changes so that the source of stress and negative emotion does not recur. It takes time for the physical, emotional, mental and spiritual bodies to be brought back into balance.

The Human Energy System:

The human body consists of a physical body as well as an energy body. The subtle body consists of prana (energy), the aura, the chakras and the nadis.

Prana

Prana is the universal principal of energy. It is the life force. It is the life force in which all of life is based from. It is described as our inner power and strength, breath, respiration, our spiritual essence. It is a complex phenomenon with its nature being highly changeable and constantly moving. It is often related to a current of electricity, constantly flowing and pulsating. Prana flows and pulsates through our bodies through "nadis" (called in Sanskrit) or "meridians" (called in Chinese medicine). These highways of energy can often become blocked, stagnated, over-stimulated or simply imbalanced. When this occurs, toxins are produced and disease settles into the body. It is important to become consciously aware of prana so we can manipulate, harness and channel it for greater degrees of awareness.

Chakras

There are seven main chakras located along the spinal column, which are energy centers of the body. These chakras are like spirals of energy, each one relating to the others and they feed universal energy to all the body systems and functions. Each chakra vibrates at a specific vibration frequency and resonates with a specific color, sound, life lesson, emotional state and thought. When these centers are balanced, one's life becomes more balanced both physically and emotionally. The word chakra derives from Sanskrit and means "wheel" or "turning".

The 7 Main Chakras

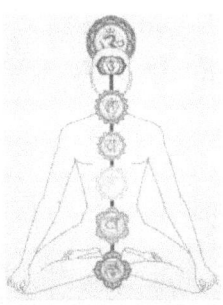

7th Chakra Sahasrara / Crown Chakra

6th ChakraAjna / Third eye Chakra

5th ChakraVishuddhi / Throat Chakra

4th ChakraAnahata / Heart Chakra

3rd ChakraManipura / Navel – Solar Plexus Chakra

2nd ChakraSwadhistana / Sacral Chakra

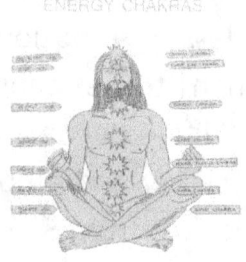

1st ChakraMuladhara / Root Chakra

1st Chakra

ROOT CHAKRA/ MULADHARA	
LOCATION	BASE OF SPINE

GLAND	ADRENAL
SYSTEM	EXCRETORY, MUSCLE, SKELETON
ORGAN	KIDNEYS, BLADDER, SPINAL COLUMN, LEGS
FUNCTION	KUNDALINI, SECURITY, GROUNDING, FEAR, PHYSICAL ENERGY
COLOUR	RED
ELEMENT	EARTH
MANTRA	LAM

2nd Chakra

SACRAL CHAKRA/ SWADHISTAN	
LOCATION	BELOW NAVEL
GLAND	GONADS
SYSTEM	REPRODUCTIVE SYSTEM
ORGAN	SEX ORGANS
FUNCTION	ANGER, ACTION, SEXUALITY, PEACE

COLOUR	ORANGE
ELEMENT	WATER
MANTRA	YAM

3rd Chakra

SOLAR PLEXUS/ MANIPURA CHAKRA

LOCATION	STOMACH TREE INCHES ABOVE THE NAVEL
GLAND	PANCREAS
SYSTEM	DIGESTIVE SYSEM
ORGAN	LIVER, STOMACH, GALL BLADDER, LARGE INTESTINE, SPLEEN
FUNCTION	EMOTION, POWER, WISDON, ACTION
COLOUR	YELLOW
ELEMENT	FIRE
MANTRA	RAM

4th Chakra

HEART CHAKRA/ ANAHATA

LOCATION	HEART
GLAND	THYMUS
SYSTEM	**CIRCULATORY SYSTEM, VAGUS NERVE, ARMS**
ORGAN	**HEART, LUNGS, BLOOD, LIVER, COMPASSION, LIFE FORCE**
FUNCTION	**GROUP, CONSCIOUSNESS, LOVE**
COLOUR	**GREEN (GRASS)**
ELEMENT	AIR
MANTRA	YAM

5th Chakra

THROAT CHAKRA/ VISHUDDHI

LOCATION	THROAT
GLAND	THYROID
SYSTEM	**LYMPHATIC SYSTEM**

ORGAN	THROAT, UPPER LUNGS, ALIMENTARY CANAL, BRONCHIAL & VOCAL APPARATUS
FUNCTION	COMMUNICATION, SELF EXPRESION, CREATIVE ENERGY, SOUND
COLOUR	SKY BLUE
ELEMENT	ETHER
MANTRA	HUM

6th Chakra

BROWN CHAKRA/ AJNA	
LOCATION	FOREHEAD BETWEEN EYE BROW
GLAND	PITUITARY
SYSTEM	AUTONOMIC NERVOUS SYSTEM
ORGAN	HYPOTHALAMUS, LOWER BRAIN, SPINE, LEFT EYE, NOSE, EARS
FUNCTION	THIRD EYE, INTUITION, CLAIRVOYANCE, INTELLIGENCE, LIGHT, TELEPATHY

COLOUR	INDIGO
ELEMENT	ETHER
MANTRA	UNIVERSAL SOUND- OM

7th Chakra

CROWN CHAKRA/ SAHASTRAR	
LOCATION	TOP OF THE HEAD
GLAND	PINEAL
SYSTEM	CEREBRO SPINAL NERVOUS SYSTEM
ORGAN	UPPER BRAIN, RIGHT EYE
FUNCTION	SPIRITUAL VISION ENLIGHTMENT
COLOUR	VIOLET
ELEMENT	ETHER
MANTRA	UNIVERSAL SOUND- OM

Aura

The aura is the electromagnetic field that surrounds the human body and every organism and object in the universe. There are seven layers of human aura, which are corresponding with the seven chakras. The layers are called etheric body, emotional body, mental body, astral body, etheric template body, celestial body and etheric/causal body. These layers of energy are suspended around the healthy human body in an oval shaped field. This "auric egg" emits out from the body approximately 2-3 feet on all sides. It extends above the head and below the feet into the ground. Each one of the subtle bodies that exist around the physical body, have its own unique color and frequency, they are interrelated and affect one another and the person's feelings, emotions, thinking, behavior and health as well. Therefore a state of imbalance in one of the bodies leads to a state of imbalance n the others.

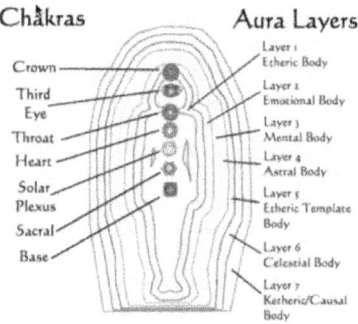

Nadis

Nadi in Sanskrit derives from the word nad with means flow. They are known in the Chienese medicine as Meridians. Nadis are the energy channels of the body and there are approximately 72'000 of them in the subtle body and connected by the chakras, which charges the nadis. The chakras function as valves, regulating the flow of prana (energy). Through the nadis and chakras the prana is delivered to every cell of the body and this is enhanced through the breath.

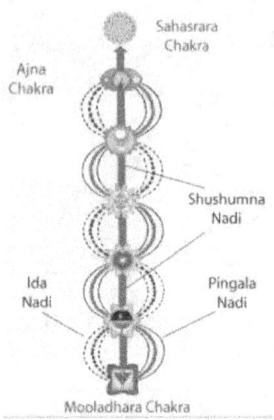

The 3 major nadis that connect the main chakras together are called Ida, Pingala and Sushumna.

Ida represents the female, Yin, cooling energy. It relates to the right brain hemisphere, creativity, making us caring, loving, emotional and giving inspiration, vision, imagination. Starting at the third eye region, coming out through the left nostril, governing the left nasal passage.

Pingala is the male, dominant energy, it is Yang in nature, heating, rational, relating to the Sun. It is the motivation that moves us forward, the determination in us, independence and pride. Left brain functioning, logic and linearity goes with it. Pingala also starts at the third eye and its aperture point is the right nostril, giving prana to the right nasal passage.

Sushumna is the central nadi, our "astral spine", hidden along and in our physical spine, relating to our central nervous system is controlling the functioning of all our chakras on the subtle level. Its energy flow is very limited, or blocked, till you achieve such an inner-outer balance in your being, with various yogic practices, that the Kundalini-Shakti Energy of Super Consciousness can freely flow up from the Muladhara, our Root Chakra, where she is said to be waiting coiled like a snake three and a half times.

The other two (Ida &Pingala) of the three important ones are the energies of opposites. They spiral around the central nadi, creating our main energy centers at their crossing points, merging into One at the Third Eye.

Chapter 6: Hand Placement For Healing Yourself

And so we begin using the art of reiki to heal yourself. Because the universe's life force is flowing through everyone and everything at all times, using reiki on yourself does not require any special effort or particular choreography. The art of reiki treatments are simply to place your hands on certain parts of your body in order to allow the energy to move and flow between the two touching places. Remember, the energy is already there. The energy is already flowing. You are simply attempting to direct it. You are simply attempting to channel it. You are not the energy. You are simply a conduit and our attempting to make it flow more freely in particular areas.

The way you go about channeling energy is by putting your hands in specific positions on your own body. You do not need any special knowledge about anatomy. Nor do you need to know exactly what part of your own body is most in need. The universal energy is omnipotent and all-knowing. The life force will move to where it is most needed on its own. There is no right or wrong way to place your hands upon yourself. These are simply suggestions and can be modified or experimented with at any time, especially upon yourself.

There are 10 different general hand placements that we will discuss using on yourself:

Face

Head

Neck

Chest

Stomach

Shoulders

Back

Hips

Legs

Feet

Face

Much like if you were washing your face with your hands place your palms over your face, your fingers over your eyes, your eyes closed and breathe. Move your hands up, caressing your fingertips over your forehead to the top of your hairline and bringing your hands down along the side of your face, letting your fingertips move down around your temples, feeling over your cheekbones, down to where your jawline starts and across to the middle of your chin. Bring your fingertips to your nose, letting the flat pads of your fingers lay against your cheeks and bring your hands around in a small circle letting your fingertips end up on your lips. Feel free to continue moving your hand around your face, or simply letting your hands lay still on your face. Because our faces and the skin in this area is so sensitive, please take care to do everything very gently. Make sure your eyes are closed. Be sure to not poke yourself in the eye. Go as slowly as you need.

Let your fingers come back to your jaw bone where it meets your neck, and lay one hand along each side of your jaw. Feel the curve of your jaw bone in the palm of your hand. Then slowly but firmly press your fingertips into your jaw bone and gently drag your fingers down to your chin. Turning your fingers to face towards your ears and bringing your wrists together to touch at your chin, simply rest your hands on your jaw. Now cross your arms and place your right hand over your left jaw bone and your left hand over your right jaw bone, repeating the previous movement of your fingers down to your chin.

2. Head

Cupping your hands over your ears and moving your hands towards your face half an inch, let your fingers rest around your temples. Bring your hands toward the top of your head, letting your pinkies lineup along your hairline. Gently let your hands fall down and around the back of your head, as if you were rinsing water out of your hair. Clasp your fingers around each other at the base of your skull, letting your head rest in your hands for a moment. Then unlock your fingers and bring your hands back up to just behind your ears. Again, feel free to go as slowly as necessary. You may or may not want to use more pressure on your scalp. Feel free to use your fingertips to get beneath the hair and to the skin on your head, although this is not necessary. Take care while placing your hands on your head not to move your neck too much. You do not need to move your neck to reach any places in particular. You also do not want to strain your neck doing this.

3. Neck

Very gently place one hand over the front of your neck, making sure not to apply any pressure or squeeze whatsoever. Feel your pulse underneath your finger. Gently put your other hand on the back of your neck, allowing your fingers to touch around your neck if possible. If not possible, do not force this. It is not necessary. Release your hands and turning your fingers toward your ears place both of your hands on either side of your neck, with your wrists touching in front of you, just underneath your chin. Release and cross your arms in front of you, allowing your right hand to wrap around the left side of your neck and your left hand to wrap around to the right side of your neck.

Now allow your hands to continue traveling down your neck and across your collarbone. Feel your décolletage extend out to your shoulders. Then bring your hands back across to the opposite side allowing your left hand to end up on your left shoulder and your right hand to end up on your right shoulder, if that is possible for you. If you cannot reach or are not flexible enough to touch your shoulders, that is quite all right.

4. Chest

Laying each hand on the top of your chest just below the collarbone, keep your hand flat, but do not apply pressure or push down on your chest. As much as you are comfortable feel free to move your hands across your chest. Make sure to place at least one hand right between your breasts, as this is where the heart chakra resides. Move your hands down further and place each palm over either side of your rib cage. Allow your hands to fall down the sides of you as far as is comfortable for your flexibility. Then cross your arms and place your right hand over your left rib cage and your right hand over your left rib cage starting from your far side moving your hands in toward each other meeting at the center of your chest. With your fingertips, drag your fingers up your center chest towards your neck and back down, using just your fingertips.

Because your chest takes up a wide swath of your body, feel free to spend as much or as little time here as you would like. Using your hands to go up and down the center of your chest repeatedly is a good practice that you will find has a lot of soothing qualities.

5. Stomach

Laying your hands on your stomach, this is another area that will do well with up and down emotions over the center of your stomach. The stomach will also benefit from using circular motions, specifically clockwise motions over your digestive system. It is especially helpful to make tracks across your stomach from side-to-side two or three times. You can do this in many ways. You can put both hands next to each other, side-by-side, starting on your left side and dragging both of your hands across your stomach over the middle and down to your right side, and then going back from right to left. You can do this two or three times. Or you could start with one hand on each side, and simultaneously move them toward each other and then across to the opposite side. Again, going back and forth two or three times.

However, some people find this to be uncomfortable, especially after having eaten. In that case, feel free to simply lay your hands statically on your stomach, without movement. Another great exercise to do here is by letting your middle fingers touch each other tip-to-tip, and laying those right over your navel. Let your hands lay here, right over the center of your stomach for a few moments. No movement is necessary.

6. Shoulders

If you are lying down, you may want to sit up or stand in order to do your shoulders.

Reaching up and over your own shoulders as much as is comfortable for your level of flexibility, place your hands on your shoulders and run them as far down your back as possible. With your hands on your back, run your hands back and forth from side to side, applying as much pressure with your fingertips as you would like. Release your hands, cross your arms in front of you, and place each hand on the opposite shoulder feel free to reach as far behind you as possible, although this may be very difficult. Move your hands over your shoulders and down your arms ending up with your hands holding each other. You can also take one arm at a time to reach the back of your shoulder blades. Lifting your right arm straight above you, bend at the elbow so that your hand is now behind your head. Put your left hand on your right elbow and allow it to push your right hand farther down your back. Again, this is important to note that you should not do anything that hurts or is uncomfortable. You do not need to reach farther down your shoulder blades then is comfortable for you.

7. Back

To reach your back, you can simply place your hands behind your back, and use either the back of your hands if that is all that is feasible for you based on your flexibility, or if you are able to turn your palms towards your back, even for just a small portion of area, you can do that as well. In your back, a great motion would be going up and down your spine, making sure not to apply any pressure, and repeating this motion a few times. The same as with your stomach, you can also move your hands back and forth from side to side across your back as much as is possible for you. An important area to try to reach on your back would be your low back area. Placing your right hand on your right low back and your left hand on your left low back, allowing your fingertips to point towards your buttocks, let your hands rest here for a moment over your root chakra.

8. Hips

From there you can simply move your hands further down to rest on your hip bones. As always, do whatever is most comfortable for you, because this is simply for yourself. Move your hands further back as far as you can feel your hip bones around you, and is comfortable for your amount of flexibility. Moving your hands back and forth over your hip bones two or three times. Move your hands lower about one inch in order to feel the very top of the leg where it connects to your hip. Again move your hands back and down as far as comfortable for you. Then turn your wrists as much as possible pointing your fingertips down toward your toes and move your hands from side to side. Much like with your stomach, you can do this a couple of ways. Placing your hand side by side and moving from left to right together, or starting with one hand on either side and crossing opposite of each other.

9. Legs

While performing reiki on yourself, this is the point at which if you were laying, you will most likely need to sit up. You could also always perform it on yourself while sitting in a chair. In order for you to reach your own legs, get into whatever position is most comfortable for you. Placing your hands on the top of your thighs, feel free to move your hands up, down, and all around your upper legs. Make sure to take turns using the opposite hand on the opposite leg. It is best to take some time using both hands on your left leg, as well as using both hands on your right leg. As much as possible based on how you are sitting, standing, or laying, reach as much as possible to feel the underside of your thighs, as well.

Next you will move to your own knees. Feel free to cup one hand over each knee and move it around in a circular motion. Again, make sure to use your right hand on your left knee and your left hand on your right knee as well. This helps to move energy across your body. While you are at your knee, cup both hands around each knee for a moment. Then use your left hand on your right knee and your right hand on your right hip in order to channel energy from these two areas of major movement. After a moment, be sure to switch, with your right hand on your left knee and your left hand on your left hip.

Moving your hands down your calf, again going as slowly as you need and crossing your hands over to the opposite side as well as using both hands on each side. Do the same as you just did for your knee and hip you should do with your knee and ankle. Putting your left hand on your right ankle and your right hand on your right knee, pause here for a moment. Release and switch to do the same on the other side.

10. Feet

For your feet, because they contain so many bones and so much energy, even though they may seem small, you will want to take the time to truly cover all of your feet. Placing your palms on the top of your foot and moving it down towards your toes, and then back up again towards your ankle a few times. You will also want to lay your palms flat on the top of your feet moving your hands from side to side across the width of your foot from your pinky toe to your big toe and down over the arch of your foot and bringing your fingertips around your ankle back to your heel. You can use slight pressure with your fingertips if it is comfortable, if not there is no need. Starting with your fingertips on your toes drag your hands back across the sides of your feet and back around your ankle, cupping your heel. Lifting your foot up, place your flat palm against the bottom of your foot, moving your hand up and down. Wrap your palm around your toes moving your hand back and forth across all of your toes. Cup the bottom of your heel into your hand rotating your hand around in a circular motion. Using both of your hands cup either side of your ankle and rotate your hands as much as possible around your ankle.

Chapter 7: Creating A Healing Partnership.

Cats are very energy-sensitive, especially to feelings of anger, stress, and unhappiness that may be exhibited by their human companions. It is essential, however, that you find a way to reach a state of personal relaxation and inner peace when you offer a Reiki treatment to your cat. Doing so creates a safe, comfortable environment that your cat will recognize and gravitate towards so you can assist them through their healing journey.

Meditation is an excellent pathway to reach a peaceful state of mind prior to offering a Reiki treatment. The following meditation is based on the Reiki Principles re-stated as one-word affirmations combined with five special Reiki hand positions that I developed. Each hand position is held for 2-3 minutes while you softly chant the appropriate affirmation.

The meditation takes only 10-15 minutes to complete and should be done in any quiet place where you can sit or lie down comfortably and not be disturbed. The practice of this meditation on a regular basis will greatly help you reach a state of relaxation and peace.

MY REIKI MEDITATION

· Sit or lie down, close your eyes, and take several deep-cleansing breaths.

· Pace both your hands (palms down) gently over your eyes and chant the word "CALM" for 2-3 minutes.

- Place your dominant hand on your forehead and your other hand on the back of your head. Chant the word "SERENITY" for 2-3 minutes.

- Keep your dominant hand on your forehead and move your other hand to your navel (about 2 inches below your belly button). Chant the word "COMPASSION" for 2-3 minutes.

- Move your dominant hand to your throat while keeping your other hand on your navel. Chant the word "INTEGRITY" for 2-3 minutes.

- Move your dominant hand to cover your heart and keep your other hand on your navel. Chant the word "GRATITUDE" for 2-3 minutes.

- Conclude with several deep-cleansing breaths before you open your eyes.

INTRODUCING YOURSELF AND REIKI TO A CAT:

Always respect a cat's personal space when you introduce yourself for the first time. If you are wearing sunglasses or a hat, remove them. Sit in a low chair or on the ground at least 5 feet away from the cat.

Slowly drop your arms to your side with your hands turned downwards and palms facing forward. Speak quietly and reassuringly to the cat and avoid direct eye contact. Do not make any sudden movements. If you are meeting the cat for the first time, softly introduce yourself and that you are there to OFFER the cat healing energy that is gentle, safe, and very relaxing.

Let the cat decide how much, if any, energy that it is willing to accept. The cat will display its comfort level with the treatment with its body language. Visual signs of acceptance include displays of:

· Direct eye contact.

· Pushing its head or body into your hands.

- Lying down on or very near you.
- Drooping its eyelids, drooling, or falling asleep.
- Licking or smelling your hands.
- Deep sighing, yawning, or purring.

If the cat chooses to reject the energy treatment, it will likely display that response by:

- Moving or turning away from you (however, if the cat remains nearby, it is accepting the energy and revealing to you where it would like it directed).
- Constantly pacing around or by leaving the area.
- Making growling or hissing noises.
- Lashing its tail or by laying its ears back against its head.

A cat's body reveals quite a bit about the mood of the cat; below is some additional cat body language to look for:

- **Whiskers:**

- Straight out to the sides = a happy and relaxed cat.

- Flattened back against its nose = a fearful or angry cat.

• **Ears:**

- Perked up and slightly forward = a happy and friendly cat.

- Straight back against its head = an annoyed, angry, or frightened cat.

- Swiveling around to the outside = a curious cat.

· Tails (posture and movement):

- Between its legs = an fearful and submissive cat.

- Straight up = a happy, friendly, playful cat.

- Fluffed out and up = an angry or upset cat.

- Fast twitching tip or tail lashing back and forth = a very irritated cat.

- Slow twitching tip = a happy, comfortable cat.

• **Eyes:**

- Wide open and dilated = a fearful cat.

- Narrowed and dilated = a very angry cat.

- Shut = a contented or tired cat.

DO YOU HAVE A NEUROTIC CAT?

The common symptoms of a neurotic cat include the following:

· Being extremely nervous around people and other pets.

· Being easily and greatly spooked by sudden noises and movements.

· Preferring to be alone, often hiding under a bed.

· Hissing or growling when being petted or picked up.

- Frequent running around like crazy for no apparent reason.

- Puffing up its fur and arching its back for no apparent reason.

- Swatting (not playfully) at people as they walk by.

- Constantly knocking items off of tables and counters.

The causes for this behavior may be due to stress from conflicts between several opposing courses of action, such as when your cat is faced with a "fight or flight" choice (i.e. your cat is inside and sees another cat in "its" yard). Or, your cat greets your return home after an extended absence (to your cat) with happy chirps followed by an angry bite or swipe of its paw. This is separation anxiety from being left alone too long or too often with no other sources of companionship, entertainment, or food to distract it. Reiki can help.

Chapter 8: Meditation Techniques To Harness The Power Of Reiki

Now that you have learned how you can use Reiki to cleanse your being, it is time to begin your Reiki meditation and choose a technique that suits you the best. There are different techniques that have developed over the years. You have the earlier techniques and the modern ones that are the result of drifts in the spiritual and religious influences on Reiki.

All the meditation techniques that are followed in Reiki follow the five elements of Reiki that you have read about in the first book. Now, there are three major techniques including Kenkyoku Ho, Joshin Ho and Seishin Toistu. The first one is a cleansing technique, the second one uses the breath to focus the mind, and the third works entirely on unifying your mind. All traditional forms of Reiki will practice these three techniques of meditation alone.

There is yet another type of meditation that is taught at the second level. This is called Hatsurei ho. It is basically a combination of the three forms of meditation that are mentioned above. There is also an original version of this meditative form that was written by Tomita Kaiji, a student of Usui. This original form of meditation was written in the year 1933.

Development of these meditative techniques

Special breathing techniques called Kokyu have long been used not only in Japanese martial arts but also most of their religious practices. Usui, the founder of Reiki was proficient in both. There are several martial arts like aikido and Jujitsu that advocate the used of these breathing techniques. They are responsible for the awareness created about these meditation techniques. These breathing techniques are believed to unify your body and mind and help you develop from within as an individual.

When Usui died in the year 1926, several meditation techniques emerged. They were taught under different systems of Reiki. They became popular in the Western world only around the late 1930s. There were several other techniques that just died out because they were not as well propagated as the traditional and also a few contemporary ones.

The traditional techniques of meditation

Mentioned below are some of the oldest and most traditional meditation practices of Reiki:

1. Hatsurei Ho

This method is mostly aimed at generating a large amount of spiritual energy. This technique is one of the earliest meditation techniques used in conjunction with Reiki. Records of this meditation technique are present in a book by Kaijo Tomita that was written as early as 1933. He was a student of Usui Mikao. There are simpler translations of this technique in several books these days. The difference between Eastern and Western practices of this technique is that in the west waka chanting is not practiced. Waka is a form of poetry that was composed by the Meiji Emperor. This is the breakdown of the meaning of this meditation technique.

Hatsu means to generate

Rei means spirit

Ho means method

To initiate this practice of meditation, you need to find a quiet room and sit still for a while focusing on the body and mind. You have two options- you can practice Reiki in a seated position or while you are performing the action of sitting.

Sitting still or sitting in seiza allows you to concentrate on the energy that you are receiving and transmitting throughout your body. This is when you can channelize the energy from your heart and mind into your palm. Keep the shoulders and arms relaxed and join the palms together. Then focus on the alignment of your body and keep your eyes closed.

When you are in this posture, it is time to purify the mind. Some utter waka poetry and others just practice breathing techniques. This allows you to put your entire focus on the mind, thereby cleansing it of any unpleasant and untoward thoughts and experiences. You will be able to find these waka poems or listen to them online.

The practice

After you have followed the aforementioned steps, you may begin to feel some warmth in your palm. According to Tomita ryu, this is reiha working on your body. Reiha is nothing but the wave of the rei energy entering your body. You will feel a tingling sensation that is almost like a mild current passing through your body. The rei and the heat that is generated are the spiritual energies that are working on you. Even if they are not as strong in the beginning, they will get better and better as you concentrate and practice more.

Make a 5-day schedule

All the methods and steps mentioned above should be practiced at least for 5 consecutive days. Make sure that you breathe or utter waka poems for at least 30 minutes each day. You may progressively increase this time to at least one hour.

2. Kenyoku Ho

This is a Japanese practice that is aimed mostly at purifying your body, spirit and heart. It is usually performed before you actually conduct a session of Reiki on another person or even yourself. You will use swift sweeping motions of the palm across your body almost as if you are taking a bath. Here is a sequence of the cleansing process that you need to practice and follow:

Make sure that you start with your shoulders. Start with your right shoulder and use your left hand to make a sweeping motion down towards the right hip. Repeat the same on the other side. Finish this off with one more sweep from the right shoulder to the right hip. Keep your left elbow against the side of your body. Let the left arm parallel to the ground, horizontally. Now, using your right hand, make a sweeping action from your left shoulder, down the arm up to the fingertips of the left hand. Repeat the same on the other side. Then, finish the process off with one more sweep on the left side while the left hand is horizontal to the floor.

With these simple meditation and cleansing practices, you should be able to strengthen your Reiki energy by several folds.

Chapter 9: Symbols

There are six different symbols that are used in the Reiki practice in Western civilization, but not all of these symbols were originally used by Usui Sensei. A few of them were invented by the people who brought Reiki to the Western part of the world. Some of them were changed due to the fact that Reiki Masters are not allowed to write down the symbols they are using. Thus, these symbols are a basic guideline for the Reiki practice.

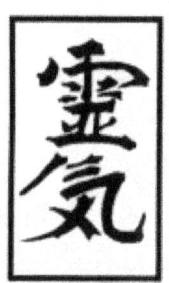

The first symbol I am going to discuss is the Reiki Symbol, it is a symbol used to communicate the word Reiki in Japanese.

This symbol was created by Usui Sensei in order to spread the word of his new practice.

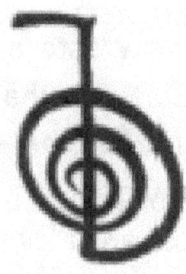

The second symbol is known as Cho Ku Ray.

This symbol is translated into 'God and man coming together'. It is primarily used to increase Reiki power and draws energy from around the user and focuses it to where the person wants it to go. If you want to use this symbol, make it over the client or yourself and silently repeat the name of the symbol three times. Uses for this symbol include:

On the spot treatments

Cleaning out negative energy

Spiritual protection

Can be used on people; water; food; medicine; and even herbs

Commonly used in sick rooms of hospitals

Aids manifestation

Empowers the other Reiki symbols to make them stronger

Seals the energies after a treatment

If you wish to bring any of these properties onto yourself, you must reverse the symbol.

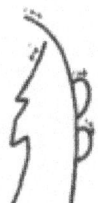

The third symbol is known as Sei Hei Ki.

It is used for mental and emotional healing. The symbol's name translates to 'God and man coming together' or 'key to the universe'. The following are its uses:

Protection of the psyche

Cleansing

Activation of kundalini in meditation

Putting a balance between the right and the left hemispheres of the brain

Aids in removing addictions

The healing of past traumas

Alignment of the upper chakras

This symbol can be used either on yourself or another while you are practicing healing.

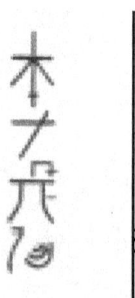

The fourth symbol is Hon Sha Ze Sho Nen.

It translates to 'the God in me greets the God in you to promote enlightenment and peace'. This is also referred to as the distance symbol for the single reason that it promotes distant healing over physical distance and time to anyone or anything.

The fifth symbol is Tam-A-Ra-Sha.

This symbol is known as the 'balancing factor' because it balances the chakras and does the unblocking of the physical; emotional; as well as mental blockages. It is a symbol well used to ground and also balance your energy; unblock your energy chakras; all this in order that your energy can flow and reduce pain; or even dissipate it when it is signed over an area in physical pain.

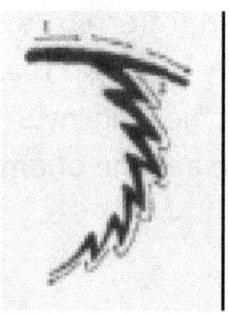

The sixth symbol is known as Dai Ko Myo.

This symbol was not created by Usui Sensei, but it is commonly used amongst the Masters of this practice. Each symbol is a little different when given to a different Master; therefore, the above is just a reference. The Master Symbol is only used by Reiki Masters to heal your soul. Still they use it to heal your spiritual self in order to heal disease, illness, and promote enlightenment and peace.

There are other symbols that are currently in practice all over the globe, but what you have here are among the main and original symbols. The Reiki symbols are simply Japanese writing. Therefore, the symbol actually stands for a word or an idea, and that is why there are numerous ones around the world.

Several methods exist for using these symbols, but none of them involve writing the symbol down or actually putting a marker to someone's body. The actual methods used with these symbols include drawing them on your palm center, drawing them with your finger, visualizing them, drawing them with your third eye, and spelling the symbol's name three times. Remember, these symbols should be used with care and are only effective when used by someone who has gone through attunement.

If you are treating only yourself, place the symbols on your palms. Then proceed with the Reiki practice. If you are using these symbols on clients, then place the symbols on the palms of your hands and redraw or visualize them on the client's crown chakra; palms; as well as the areas that require treatment. The symbols will help enhance your healing efforts.

Chapter 10: The Intricacies Of Intention Setting

Much like other ancient healing techniques, so too does reiki follow a systematic flow of steps. This pattern helps make sure that you're prepared and well-equipped throughout the entire process, guaranteeing that your mindset is appropriate and that your energy is as positive as it can be.

Just like crystal healing, the process of reiki healing also begins with an integral first step - **setting your intention**

14th Thing you need to know...

The Importance of Breaking Self Limits

Before any healing practice takes place, it's vital that you break any limitations you might have imposed on yourself or your healing capabilities. First time healers will often struggle with this, thinking that they're not **prepared or good enough** to heal themselves through reiki.

Self-doubt can be a powerful mechanism that works against your real potential. Therefore, it's best that you work away these limitations first before you engage in healing to maximize the benefits of your practice.

While it's normal for you to feel apprehensive about your capacity to heal yourself, there are things you can do to feel more confident and capable in your reiki healing power. The best way would be to **write affirmations** that reduce your self doubt and make you more trusting of the process you're about to undertake.

As the first step of your healing, take a piece of paper and a pen, and write down affirmations that make you feel more trusting of your inherent healing power. Here are some examples of affirmations that you can write down:

I am an empowered, capable child of the divine universe. I am deserving of all the positivity that life has to offer.

My heartfelt desires deserve to be fulfilled.

I am open to the gifts of the universe. My arms are spread wide to receive all the positivity that comes my way. I am receptive of these gifts and blessings.

I am capable of healing. I have the power inside of me, and this potent gift cannot be corrupted - only improved and enhanced.

As you write your affirmation, make sure to truly feel the meaning of the words. Meditate upon the words and feel the energy of the universe flowing into your system. Visualize the benefits of reiki healing and try to picture out your life after you've received these gifts. Strive to become the person in your visions and choose to trust in your inherent ability to become your own healer.

15th Thing you need to know…

Setting Your Intention

Once you feel more confident in your healing capabilities, it's time to set your intention. Your intention is basically what you want to achieve with your reiki healing practice. There is no wrong or right way to state your intention, and there is no aspect of your being that can't be made an intention. So essentially, whatever it is you feel needs healing can be set as your intention to maximize the benefits of your reiki healing practice.

Throughout the day, you probably already set intentions in some shape, way, or form. "**I hope I can finish my workload today. I wish my mom takes my pregnancy news positively. I pray my boss agrees to my request for a raise.**" All of these statements demonstrate intentions that we set for ourselves in our daily lives.

In the same way, your reiki healing intention is what you **aim to achieve** through the healing practice. By setting your intention, you can direct your effort more specifically in order to restore the flow of your life force where you might be experiencing disturbance.

16th Thing you need to know...

Specific Intentions are More Effective

The more specific you are when it comes to setting your intentions, the more effective your healing practice becomes. **Why?** Remember that the process of directing the healing energy where you want it to go will rely on your own capabilities. The more specific your intention, the more precisely you'll be able to direct the healing power to achieve the results you want.

For instance, instead of saying "I want to be pregnant someday", **opt for something more specific, like** "I will conceive by June of this year and have a healthy baby boy by March of next year."

See how it changes the energy of your intention? By being as specific as possible, it becomes easier to visualize the fruit of your reiki healing practice. And in effect, you become more capable of directing your healing energy where it needs to be for a more effective effort.

17th Thing you need to know...

Positive Intentions are Best

It's always easier to mention all the things you don't want. But by phrasing your intention in a negative way, you might also have a negative impact on the positivity of the energy you imbibe. Negative intentions create an atmosphere of dislike, dissatisfaction, and unhappiness, which may stir negative emotions as you go through the healing process.

Avoid using negative words like "don't", "won't", and "can't", and focus on more positive versions of your intentions in order to reap the maximum benefits of your healing practice. For instance, instead of saying "**I won't fall victim to the same emotional stress that my ex put me through**", opt for something more positive like, "**I will discover a genuine, pure love that will bring me greater joy and satisfaction than I've ever known.**"

18th Thing you need to know...

Always Strive for the Most

Your intention doesn't simply end with what you want for yourself. In most instances, the universe will surprise you by giving you things that exceed your own expectations. So, don't limit your intentions by adding finality. Instead, add a phrase at the end of each intention in order to maximize the potential rewards of your healing practice.

How do you do this? Adding phrases like "... or better" or "...or more" can be simple yet powerful ways to increase the potential of your intention. So, for instance, using the previous example, you might say something like "**I will discover a**

genuine, pure love that will bring me greater joy and satisfaction than I've ever known or better."

19th Thing you need to know…

Keep It Personal

Personal intentions work best because the only person you truly know is yourself. We can't control other people's fate, and neither are we responsible for other people's wellness. Only they will understand what they want and need in life, so it's best that you keep other people out of your intentions.

For instance, a mother might say "**I want my daughter to become the best in her class.**" But because her daughter's energy is disconnected from her own life force system, it might be impossible to achieve that intention.

Instead, try to focus on yourself and what you can do to have a positive impact on other people in your life. For instance, the above intention can be rephrased to "**I will**

become a supportive, understanding, and empathetic mother so that my daughter will have the guidance and love she needs in order to succeed."

If you're trying to heal someone else with your energy, avoid setting intentions for them. Instead, give them the basic principles of proper intention setting and then ask them to formulate their own intention.

20th Thing you need to know...

The Process of Setting

Now that you know the intention you want to work with, it's time that you actually set the intention. So how do you do that? For some, more experienced reiki healers who are attuned with their healing power, simply uttering the intention like a mantra during meditation can be more than enough for them to be able to direct their energy.

But if you're just starting out, then you might want to consider writing your intention down. There is a unique power to writing an intention, making it easier to visualize your end goal. As a beginner, it works best to write your intention on a slip of paper before starting the healing process in order to better focus your energy and achieve the results you're aiming for.

Take a clean sheet of paper and meditate on the intention you want to focus on. Once you've decided on how best to phrase your intention, write it down on your paper while wording it out. After you've written it, take the paper in your hands and read the intention a few times to yourself until it feels like you've fully absorbed its essence.

As you read your intention, visualize the energy of reiki flowing from the environment around you, towards the words on the paper. Charge your intention and sense the power of reiki blessing the words you've written.

Now that the intention is fully realized and properly set, you can begin the process of healing.

Chapter 11: Developing Your Reiki Practice

The least complex meaning of Reiki is that it is a "Japanese system for stress decrease and unwinding that additionally advances healing."1

Exact and straightforward, I observe that it is normally an adequate response for the vast majority. Be that as it may, Reiki is a major subject, and the above definition is a modest portrayal of the genuine way of Reiki. Understanding Reiki and the capacity to portray its profundities is a piece of the excursion. Reiki will listen to your inquiries and show you naturally. As you add to your association with Reiki, the answers you get will influence your life, convictions, needs and aims, while they help you characterize your comprehension and practice of Reiki making it into something that is remarkably your own.

A standout amongst the most well-known inquiries my understudies ask after their Reiki attunements is the means by which to discuss Reiki to others. What individuals think they think about Reiki vitality from having read about it or having gotten a Reiki treatment is altogether different than their experience after their attunements? They all of a sudden understand that there are few words to depict the manifestly obvious vitality coursing through their body. It is frequently outside what they think, opening an unforeseen field of conceivable outcomes. They discover they have no words to clarify it.

I offer recommendations about some normally examined Reiki subjects with the goal that you can arrange your considerations around how you characterize your own Reiki practice. I will offer knowledge into the profound way of Reiki and the significance of characterizing your heart aim for your Reiki practice alongside making proposals on the most proficient method to utilize Reiki to mend a percentage of the difficulties and impediments you may experience around these points. Resulting articles will talk about approaches to characterize Reiki for the medicinal group, how to characterize your requirements for Reiki and how to characterize an expert Reiki business.

Truly, we realize that Reiki advanced and was practiced by requirements of the individuals utilizing it. Usui Sensei, the author, was a profound researcher. History lets us know that he started his instruction in a Tendai Buddhist school at age four. He mulled over Buddhism, Christianity, Shinto, the enchantment of pixies, the investigation of divination and restorative science, and he fit in with a gathering devoted to creating psychic capacities.

Usui Sensei was a profound man who depended on his instinct and inward sensitivities when giving Reiki sessions. He utilized his Three Pillars of Reiki in his recuperating sessions: Gassho reflection, Reiji-Ho and Chiryo. Dr. Hayashi was a therapeutic specialist and a chief in the naval force who utilized Reiki as a typical restorative practice on board ships. Hayashi Sensei made a Reiki manual with institutionalized medications for specific physical illnesses. To suit the western world, she rolled out numerous improvements to the practice of Reiki, and at one point even painted over the word Reiki on her business sign, transforming it to "Short Wave Therapy."[2]

Yet with every one of the augmentations and changes to Reiki after Usui Sensei's practice, all still concur that it adjusts its recuperating vitality to the condition existing apart from everything else.

We see from Takata Sensei's case that Reiki recuperates paying little respect to what it is called. It is likely that you will characterize Reiki in different courses relying upon whom you are conversing with. I show Reiki with profound dialect in my Reiki classes; be that as it may, when I am in therapeutic settings I pick a great deal more unbiased dialect to portray it. This is splendidly adequate since Reiki is assorted and versatile to all convictions about it.

How to Become a Reiki Master

The right way for how to turn into a Reiki expert can depend to an expansive degree on your inspirations. What is your arrangement once you have accomplished the objective? Would you like to set up a Reiki practice? Would you like to utilize Reiki for recuperating? Would you like to thusly educate others? Then again are you most keen on the individual advantages, for example, enhanced self-acknowledgment?

It just bodes well that different procedures for how to turn into a Reiki expert may be fitting relying upon how you plan to utilize and apply this grand instrument for vitality mending and self-acknowledgment!

In reality, numerous individuals neglect the self-acknowledgment advantages of Reiki. While numerous perceive that it is connected with vitality mending, the conceivable outcomes for inward adjust and awareness ought not be reduced.

Options For How To Become A Reiki Master

After that, you can assess the different methodologies and locate the particular case that best matches your own inclinations, your learning style, and your goals!

Customarily, individuals got preparing in Reiki by adjusting to a Reiki expert. There was a procedure of working through the three levels of Reiki, with attunements occurring at every stage.

These attunements to Reiki must be performed under the direction of the expert, and just an expert is qualified to perform them.

Numerous experts concocted long courses for every level. These are a bit much, but rather from a business point of view they seemed well and good. To be sure, by means of this methodology turning into a Reiki maser can cost near to $10,000. What's more, it can take a couple of years!

Those time gauges and expense appraisals speak to the compelling. There are likewise weekend workshops which you can go to, basically finishing a lever for each weekend, with the goal that you can be qualified and ensured in three weekends.

None of this prepares you for running a practice from an organization or business viewpoint. Be that as it may, it does get you qualified as a Reiki expert. You can then independently add to the business aptitudes required for achievement!

There are likewise online procedures for how to turn into a Reiki expert. Despite the fact that these were at first glared upon by conventional bosses, without a doubt the great ones were produced by exceptionally experienced experts who needed to have the capacity to achieve a more extensive group of onlookers.

You see there are two schools of thought among the Reiki world class. Some accept that it ought to be elite and firmly controlled. Others need to spread the workmanship to however many individuals as could be expected under the circumstances.

One of the enormous advantages of the online Reiki courses is that you get the opportunity to finish them at your own particular pace. The other real point of preference is that they are a great deal less costly than the more conventional methodologies.

At long last, some of them join business and organization preparing too, with the goal that you are completely prepared for running your practice.

Reiki is one of the, if not the most intense recuperating technique for them all. Numerous individuals acquainted with it are pondering that how might they be able to turn into a Reiki expert. Here I will expose the mysteries of turning into a Reiki expert without spending all your well-deserved cash.

The truth of the matter is that the considerable mending forces of Reiki as of now lie inside you, they simply should be stirred. A hefty portion of the Reiki educators swear for the sake of taking parcels and bunches of exceptionally costly Reiki expert instructor courses, however they are off-base! You don't have to burn through several dollars to turn into a man that can ace these awesome recuperating forces.

There is truly no requirement for anyone hoping to ace Reiki to take these courses in light of the fact that the forces are there officially, in that spot inside you, inside every one of us. The main thing that you have to do is to wake those recuperating forces, large portions of the Reiki instructors have officially conceded that it isn't important to take every one of those costly courses to turn into an expert of Reiki.

A percentage of the best Reiki instructors have understood that the most effortless path for the normal individual to learn Reiki is by doing it in their own security. This is much why they have created online Reiki expert courses that pretty much anyone can take.

There are three noteworthy favorable circumstances of doing this from the security you could call your own home.

Firstly, it will cost you just a small amount of what it would in the event that you did it the conventional way. Furthermore, thusly you will ace Reiki a ton speedier than you would by taking a course on occasion and thirdly, you will get the opportunity to focus on it 100%, since you have all out genuine feelings of serenity in the protected environment you could call your own home.

Chapter 12: Western / Traditional Reiki - Difference?

There are two main schools of Reiki healing practice. These are the Western Reiki style, and Traditional Japanese Reiki. In this chapter, we will discuss the differences and similarities between the two.

Western Reiki

This is the most common form of Reiki practice today. Its origin comes from Hawayo Takato, who learned Reiki from Chujiro Hayashi, a direct student of Mikao Usui. Hawayo Takata's style of Reiki has become very successful, helping millions of people across the globe. She focuses mainly on the healing element of Reiki. In fact, her first line of experience with Reiki came from being able to heal herself after falling victim to some potentially fatal health problems. Naturally, then, as a Reiki practicioner, she would focus on healing potential.

Over time, there has been many additions to western Reiki practice. It first had its significant shift from traditional Reiki when it became adopted as a Tibetan healing practice. The practice was passed on by the cousin of Takata, Iris Ishikuro, who made the path to becoming a Reiki master much more accessible. This caused Takata's style of Reiki to spread all over the rest of the world.

Presently, western Reiki still focuses more on the process of healing as well as one's hand positions and attunement. There is also a focus on the chakras, the concept of which is Indian in origin. Western Reiki also makes use of guided meditation. This is the style of Reiki that is familiar to most.

Traditional Japanese Reiki

Mikao Usui, the original father of Reiki arrived at his discovery after spending his life in meditation, practicing martial arts and Tendai Buddhism. His main goal in creating Reiki was to use it as a path to enlightenment. He was believed to be a descendant of Samurais, and his practice of Reiki was more synonymous with being a life style. A Reiki practitioner would be expected to change his or her life and begin to live in a balanced way. In fact, Mikao is quoted as saying, "If you cannot heal yourself, how can you heal others."

Traditional Reiki uses a Japanese system of energy, which focuses on the Hara. It also includes five components, which are intertwined. In this form om Reiki practice, the meditations are traditional and often include the use of breathing techniques which help you to access energy directly from the Hara, which is its source. Practitioners of this style of Reiki often feel the energy channeling through themselves at once.

In traditional Japanese Reiki, the symbols and mantras represent two different things. The symbols are perceived as training wheels, so to speak. Once you have been able to form a connection with the energy that they represent, you do not nee to use them anymore. Mantras in Japanese Reiki are practiced in the style of Buddhism. They are chanted in order to create a vibration or sound that has healing properties.

Whereas in western Reiki, attunement is commonly practiced once, in traditional Japanese Reiki, it is done as many times as needed in order strengthen the energy of the practitioners. The five principles of Reiki are very important in this practice style and a Reiki practitioner is expected to meditate on them and live according to them from day to day.

The style of Reiki that you choose to practice depends on what you think fits your lifestyle and which your are drawn to.

Chapter 13: The Importance Ofinitiation

Size

Reiki is an approach to utilize the vitality in your grasp to adjust and revive the existence power vitality inside you. At the point when our life power vitality is high, we are less inclined to become ill. Numerous individuals who have been sick have profited by physical, mental and passionate heling from this hands-on vitality treatment. Through Reiki attunements, you can figure out how to take advantage of the existent power vitality and renew and mend yourself as well as other people. For some, the attunement or commencement procedure begins in 1st Degree Reiki Practitioners Healing Training. For other people, it is the formal commencement into mending others performed at the Reiki ace level. This book examines the job of attunement in Levels 1, 2 and Masters Reiki preparing.

With numerous reports in the media about vitality mending, more individuals are interested and looking for an introduction to vitality recuperating. Standard Reiki attunements is a demonstrated method to guarantee long haul great health. One of the attractions of Reiki is that anybody can figure out how to utilize it. Reiki bosses mend by widespread vitality or Qi, through the palms. This life renewing vitality practice is passed on from ace to student.

Reiki doesn't just treat physical wellbeing yet in addition enthusiastic, mental and otherworldly health. Ensuring your life power vitality is adjusted is the most ideal approach to guarantee all-encompassing wellbeing. This Japanese healing strategy is progressively being utilized by Western countries as a component of the mending process. Thus, request is expanding for prepared experts who can perform Reiki attunements.

Solution to choosing Reiki Initiation Master

Picking the privilege of a Reiki expert is essential to the achievement of your attunements in every one of the three degrees of training. Since Mikao Usui created Reiki in 1922, numerous varieties have pursued. Request that your planned educator clarifies their preparation and experience utilizing Reiki. Ask them to discuss their way of thinking and how it might contrast from that of other Reiki masters. And critically, get some information about any progressions or upgrades to their Reiki program from the customary practice.

The International Center for Reiki, for instance, underlines the convention of the customary Tibetan methods as well as the Usui Reiki techniques. This program affirms to make changes in accordance with the first Reiki technique. Truth be told, there are a few ancestries of Reiki instructed in Japan today – some of them hidden and others vigorously impacted by the Western procedures. Guarantee you comprehend the Reiki procedure being offered. Specifically inquire as to why this framework is the best for you.

Functional contemplations incorporate booking. When is the class held and for how long? Weekend courses have turned out to be well known however would a weeklong retreat be better for you? Charges shift extraordinarily today among schools. To teach Reiki to other people, every one of the three levels is required. At the ace level, you will be initiated into healing others. Consider at the time, cash and different assets you will require to finish Reiki master's level.

Reiki is more physically private than many specialist understanding relationships. Ask yourself how agreeable you would lie on a table for an hour getting Reiki medication from your educator. Reiki includes opening yourself up profoundly and emotionally. If you wind up guarded or bashful, keep on talking to Reiki teachers. Assess your mood. Do you feel upbeat around this person? Does the educator make you like yourself?

Planning for the Initiation Process

Clear your calendar of all commitments. If you have a ton of work and family worry during your Reiki class, it will be more sincere to open yourself up to the vitality procedure. Try not to plan any significant get-togethers during your Reiki commencement forms, particularly those including liquor.

Sanitize your arrangement of substances. Take out caffeine, liquor, meat and sugar from your diet. Consider fasting for a couple of days.

Meditate for an hour every day. This is a significant advance that will enable you to quiet your psyche and manage your vitality stream before the exercises start. You will get more from Reiki preparing

Assuming you are now raising your vitality vibrations.

Attempt and maintain a strategic distance from unpleasant circumstances and individuals. Once more, this is to help guarantee a quiet, thoughtful attitude.

Invest more energy among nature. Another unwinding strategy is to take a stroll on a bright day. Take a walk around the recreation center or by the sea as opposed to staring at the TV.

The Reiki Attunement Process

What is Reiki Initiation?

Ace Usui got his capacity to take advantage of Reiki vitality through an otherworldly reflection. The custom of passing Reiki down from ace to understudy proceeds. Attunement is another term for Initiation, or "reiju" in Japanese. Pamela Miles, a Reiki specialist, makes a noteworthy distinction between the terms "attunement" and "inception" on her blog. Understanding the genuine significance of inception will extend your Reiki practice. Quickly, attunement is frequently characterized as the strict exchange of all-inclusive vitality from master to understudy, supplying the understudy with the capacity to turn into a healer. Though inception alludes to the start of learning discipline. Learning, as Miles notes, includes posing inquiries can be constant. Like the nonstop renewal of vitality, the professional ought to constantly build up their abilities as a vitality healer. While inception better catches the genuine plan of Reiki healing, we will keep on utilizing the famous term "attunement" here. Yet rather than considering attunement a privilege of entry as a vitality healer, attempt and think about every attunement procedure as the start of a constant learning process.

Reiki Attunement - An approach Through the Three Reiki Levels

The attunement or commencement procedure happens in every one of the three degrees of Reiki: Reiki 1, Reiki 2 and Master level. At each level the Master initiates the student with more grounded mending vitality as they move to more elevated amounts of vitality vibration.

Reiki 1 includes four commencements of the physical body. To become an affirmed level 1 Reiki expert, you will find out about the vitality meridians of the body, the Reiki hand positions and Reiki life systems; and at last how to utilize the Reiki vitality framework to heal yourself as well as other people. When this learning is effectively aced, the Level 1 Reiki attunement must be given by a Certified Reiki Master. The function often takes 20 or 30 minutes.

Reiki 2 starts the unpretentious or air body. Three Reiki images are taught – control, mental and separation. Notwithstanding the sacrosanct symbols, 2ndDegree Certified Reiki Practitioners

Training teach extra images and hand positions. A few courses will likewise show removed Reiki remedy at this stage.

The Reiki Master level initiates the understudy into instructing Reiki. The Master image is educated. A few Masters allude to this third from as the official attunement or inception form as a vitality healer. At Level 3, you will figure out how to perform Reiki attunement on others.

Separation Reiki Attunement

Numerous individuals offer the chance to get Reiki and different types of vitality mending at a distance. While some separation healers have demonstrated that they draw from an amazing vitality source, most Reiki experts don't prescribe separation mending. Episodically, many people from those utilizing separation recuperating report that the vitality isn't as solid. A few masters accept that the physical touch is basic to convey the required mending vitality. Handy contemplations incorporate challenges getting neighborhood references and joining nearby Reiki gatherings where your healer likewise has a place. In the case of preparing in Reiki or looking for mending, similar capabilities for picking a Reiki ace must be utilized.

The Reiki Ideals

Learning the Reiki procedures and going through all phases of attunement/inception is just a piece of the road toward turning into a mindful vitality healer. You should likewise maintain the good and moral norms of a Reiki vitality healers. The Reiki Ideals were created by Reiki organizer Usui Mikao. The Reiki Ideals guarantee the sound and dependable routine with regards to Reiki. They are an attestation that you are the healer and in charge of your own demonstrations of mending. The first Reiki beliefs are the following:

· The mystery specialty of welcoming bliss.

- The marvelous medication of everything being equal.

- Only for now, don't outrage.

- Try not to stress and be loaded up with appreciation.

- Dedicate yourself to your work. Be thoughtful to individuals.

- Each morning and night join your hands in prayer.

- Ask these words to your heart.

- Furthermore, serenade these words with your mouth.

Check out Usui Reiki Treatment for the improvement of body and psyche

When you have learned Reiki, the capacity to mend yourself as well as other people physically, rationally, sincerely and profoundly lasts for a lifetime. Like any learning, assuming you seek after nonstop learning – that is, continually addressing and finding out more – your Reiki mending vitality will stay solid and even more, profoundly receptive to the general vitality source. While healing others is a steady wellspring of reconnection with the vitality source, getting attunements now and again from different bosses will keep you finely sensitive to the vitality source.

Inception or attunement?

Sometime after the demise of Hawayo Takata in December 1980, "attunement" started springing up. Numerous Reiki experts presently use it only for the procedure Mrs. Takata alluded to as inception ("reiju" in Japanese).

Be sure that the inception procedure is baffling, "commencement" is entirely clear. It alludes to starting.

Inception is the procedure by which a master offers a student the capacity to rehearse. Commencement ancestry keeps the training alive and is regular in Asian profound procedures.

The procedure of inception is innately baffling; what it achieves — empowering us to rehearse — isn't.

Similarly, as the pith of training is to start once more, commencement can be rehashed. Usui offered reiju to his students each time they gathered to rehearse.

The ascent of "attunement" appears to have put a conclusion to addressing. It urged specialists to see Reiki as a specific vibration of "vitality" to which individuals should be "adjusted" to rehearse. This disarray — that one is receptive to vitality as opposed to started into training — has taken on its very own existence and is currently for the most part introduced as certainty.

In any case, it is anything but a reality. It's a conviction. What's more, if Reiki practice is predicated on conviction, it's never again a training; it turns into a religion.

When you notice it that way — which is how individuals outside the New Age people group will, in general, notice it — is it so astonishing that some religious societies are against Reiki practice?

Demystifying inception, in a manner of speaking

It's difficult to really demystify inception. Considering this fact, the procedure itself is supernatural. In any case, while the inception procedure is baffling, what it achieves is down to earth and normally unmistakable. Individuals who get a Reiki inception might possibly see something during the procedure of commencement, however I would say, they see the impact.

As a youthful Reiki ace, I committed the error maybe all new masters make: I blabbered.

After some time, I realized that my mission isn't to clarify Reiki. Or maybe, my duty as a Reiki ace is just to show understudies how to rehearse Reiki, to get them to rehearse day by day self-treatment and to give them the certainty that they really can rehearse effectively.

Is inception enough?

I realize every one of my student's needs is the inception; I, likewise, realize they don't have the foggiest idea about that. I can't anticipate that they should trust me, nor do I need them to. I need understudies to build up their very own certainty. What's more, nothing I state can make certainty the path in-class practice does.

In my First-degree classes, we move into the first of the four inceptions offered in Hawayo Takata's genealogy directly after the welcome and presentations. I, at that point, lead the understudies through their first altered Reiki self-practice. After this short introductory practice and before they open their eyes, I request that they see any little contrast between the way they feel currently contrasted with how they felt when they began.

When I've delicately driven them out of their training session, the understudies share what they saw during their first practice. I don't recall the last time somebody didn't see anything.

In any event, individuals feel more settled, increasingly focused, progressively loose — and that is not how they expected to feel sitting discreetly in a gathering of outsiders.

The procedure of commencement is innately secretive; what it achieves — empowering us to rehearse — isn't.

Reiki Initiations are here to push you to reconnect with your picked life way and to turn into a channel for this Universal Life Healing Energy. It is the establishment for your own healing in your life and a chance to pass it onto other living creatures in the hour of this major vivacious progress from the third dimensional Energy to the fifth dimensional Energy. It is a mending practice and a method for living with profound regard, sympathy and empathy for the Soul and each living being including yourself, other individuals, creatures, plants and Mother Earth.

Reiki Initiations can raise your cognizance to a more prominent level and bring understanding of your actual way and subsequently the motivation to your own picked educational experience, the significance (or certainty) of disease or a problem and learning involved. Through Reiki Initiations your own vitality is being raised, your levels of awareness and mindfulness start developing – so significant from now on, to stay aware of this approaching high fifth dimensional Energy.

SO, DO WE NEED INITIATION TO BE ABLE TO USE REIKI?

Indeed, we should be initiated by a Reiki Master Teacher, who has accurately adjusted themselves. Reiki is a high, sacred Life Healing Energy and to have the option to arrive at that level our energy and awareness should be raised. We cannot do this by ourselves, a Reiki Master should be there for us to take us through those stages. This is the way Master Usui taught his understudies. There is a significant minute in each person's life when we believe we are reconnecting with our actual self and the Holy Source that individuals call Mother/Father God.

In contrast to other recuperating expressions, Reiki is passed from ace to understudy through a Reiki attunement that allows the understudy to interfere with the all-inclusive Reiki source.

So, what is Involved for Each Reiki Attunement?

Be aware that in a Reiki level 1 attunement, students are receptive to three unique images, each speaking to an alternate part of Reiki vitality: control, mental/passionate equalization and separation healing. Every understudy gets attunements to these 3 images in four separate occasions and with every reiteration the association develops.

Therefore, the attunements for Reiki level 2 and Reiki ace are comparative in nature, yet include various images, each with an alternate importance to opening your vivacious pathways.

What feeling comes through Attunement?

Be aware that getting a Reiki attunement is a ground-breaking, profound experience, as your lively pathways are opened by a Reiki ace. This vivacious opening permits the Reiki vitality to stream uninhibitedly through your body to affect your wellbeing and the soundness of others.

The sentiment of a Reiki attunement is an individual one, yet understudies regularly report that they feel an energy through their body and shivering from their head to their toes as the Reiki vitality pathways are opened.

The opening of an attunement has the impact of enhancing other lively mending and directing pathways and understudies report that accepting an attunement causes expanded instinctive mindfulness and improves any intrinsic clairvoyant affectability.

How Do You Prepare for an Attunement?

Meanwhile, how you get ready for a Reiki attunement relies upon your very own profound practice. Opening a vigorous pathway is no light issue and keeping in mind that it's important to do anything so as to get ready to get a Reiki attunement, most understudies decide to reconnect with their own otherworldly practice before their attunement, to increase the general impacts of the attunement and amplify its transformative power.

One prescribed arrangement for planning for a Reiki attunement involves a 3-day rinse before your attunement. Abstain from eating overwhelming nourishments, limit or dispose of caffeine, sugar, tobacco or liquor. Invest your energy perusing or pondering instead of sitting in front of the TV. Endeavor to discharge negative feelings, for example outrage or desire.

These arrangements will enable you to be increasingly prepared to acknowledge the otherworldly change and urge the attunement to have significant, long haul impacts on your life and prosperity.

Does an Attunement Need to be Renewed?

When you have been sensitive to Reiki, the Reiki vitality will course through you for an incredible remainder. Your capacity to channel and move Reiki vitality stays with you, as the endowment of Reiki tails you and encourages you for an incredible remainder.

So, what Are the Benefits of Receiving Attunements Remotely?

In-person classes are regularly instructed rapidly, without much time for understudies to consolidate the data. The attunements are given as one huge mob toward the part of the arrangement, without time for the understudies to plan for the significant otherworldly change that an attunement involves. By studying remotely, you can learn and incorporate the advantages of Reiki at your own pace and take a couple of days to set yourself up for your attunement before you get it.

Reiki is a thrilling practice and a great part of the Reiki you get and convey all through a mind-blowing remainder will be a long time experience. Starting your Reiki venture remotely encourages you to get ready for an existence of Reiki without outskirts.

Chapter 14: Benefits Of Healing Energy

There are many benefits to healing energy therapy. People use healing energy to calm stress and anxiety, strengthen well-being, reduce fatigue, reduce the side effects of medication, and recover from pain. People describe it as "intensely" relaxing. Because healing energy can lessen pain and anxiety, patients begin to feel more hopeful about regaining their health and well-being. Reiki clears the mind and helps patients be more proactive about their own health.

A few medical conditions Reiki can help improve are:

- Cancer
- Heart disease
- Anxiety
- Depression
- Chronic pain

- Chronic fatigue and other fatigue syndromes
- Infertility
- Inflammatory bowel diseases
- Autism
- Neurodegenerative disorders like Parkinson's and Alzheimer's disease

Let's take a look more closely at the benefits of energy healing, and how they can improve your life.

Improve health and wellness. Because of the energy restoring benefits of Reiki, cancer, chronic illness, and previous injuries can be healed while also improving digestion and circulation. Health and wellness in a general sense are restored leading to a healthier life overall. Some other amazing health benefits of energy healing:

- Releases tension and anxiety: Reiki allows for a sacred space where we can let go of outside tension and stress and instead focus on what is going on in our bodies and minds, helping you learn how to be more present in the moment.

- Relief from and increased resistance from depression: Energy healing aids depression by increasing serotonin and endorphins in the brain, without using harmful medications such as anti-depressants and anti-anxiety medication.

- Helps the body heal itself: Reiki helps support the immune and glandular systems through deep respiration. The deep breathing that is experienced during an energy healing session enables the parasympathetic nervous system to take over, allowing the body to function in its rest phase, instead of your body always living in fight or flight mode. Your body in its rest phase is able to heal more quickly and efficiently. Reiki is also a great supplement to traditional medications and treatments, as it is gentle, non-invasive, and speeds healing.

- Reduces blood pressure: Breathing, heart rate, and blood pressure return to normal during the deep breathing of Reiki.

- Helps rid the body of addictions: Whether the addiction is alcohol, drugs, or even food, energy healing can help. Reiki and energy healing can foster healthy feelings of well-being, meditation, and reflective thinking. Energy healing also eases the physical pain of addiction. However, doctors urge that energy healing for addiction should only be used as a complementary approach used alongside conventional recovery methods.

- Relieves pain, both acute and chronic: The International Journal of Behavioral Medicine reviewed clinical trials on biofield therapies like energy healing and concluded that there is strong evidence that these therapies greatly lessen pain in general, and moderate evidence to support long-term pain relief in chronically ill or cancer patients. Energy healing also helps people with chronic illnesses better cope with their condition. Studies involving Reiki had the greatest success.

- Removes toxins from the body's detox PATHWAYS: We spend so much time in the fight/flight mode that stress causes that our bodies hold on to dangerous toxins that can make us ill. The deep breathing and shift of the parasympathetic nervous system support the body in cleansing itself of these toxins and the negative effects they have on your energy flow.

- Increased energy and vitality to help slow the aging process: Reiki and meditation have been shown to slow down the aging process in the brain (which in turn helps with dementia). Daily stress produces free radicals (unstable atoms that attack our DNA), which makes us age much quicker. Free radicals in the body hamper the free flow of energy, which can be reversed with Reiki, thus helping us live longer, happier lives.

- Aids sleep: The biggest outcome of an energy healing session is relaxation. When we give our mind, body, and spirit time to let go and relax, we are better able to sleep at night since we are not tossing and turning with anxiety and worry.

Release bad habits and behaviors. Energy healing helps us tap into the root of negative habits and behaviors that cause them. Finding the root cause of these behaviors helps us release them, thus enabling a stronger flow of energy.

Achieve goals. Energy healing provides mental clarity, allowing us to let go of emotions that hamper us from succeeding, like feelings of inadequacy, fear, and guilt. This freeing of the mind allows for a success mentality that helps us succeed and build self-esteem. Since Reiki helps us be more present in the moment, you are less likely to get caught up in feelings of regret about the past or fear of the future, thus allowing us to "seize the day and accomplish more of our goals.

Live peacefully. Reiki and other forms of energy healing help ease depression and anxiety, replacing this stress and pent-up anger with feelings of joy and serenity. Feeling this peace and tranquility in our daily lives also aids us in feeling more compassionate towards others, which leads to kindness, an integral principle of Reiki.

Find purpose. Energy healing gives us strong feelings of meaning and purpose by restoring the flow of our chi. Opening the flow of energy allows us to listen to our intuition, which will guide us toward positive outcomes in all aspects of our lives.

The benefits of energy healing are multifold and are different for each person. Focusing on the areas you need to heal is a great way to get the benefits you are looking for. The great thing about energy healing is you can take control over your healing while you work with your healer.

Chapter 15: Reiki Attunement

What is Attunement and Why it is Essential for Reiki

Attunement is an important part of Reiki, and the basis or foundation of how a practitioner receives the energy they need to perform healing through the practice of Reiki attunement is a transference of energy from the original master to students who learn through many years of lineage and channeling energy.

The term for attunement is Reiju, which is a spiritual ritual that opens the channels of the body, through the chakras, to allow the flow of energy from the universe to enter.

The entire purpose if practicing Reiki is to clear and blockage or hindrance preventing the free flow of energy into the body.

Once these blockages are clear, the ability to transfer Reiki becomes powerful and more effective than before.

How does the attunement occur?

This is done through a ritual where the Reiki master uses a combination of symbols and mantras to connect with the students; then they transfer the universal life force to them through a specific procession.

It is important to note that every Reiki master will vary in how they conduct the attunement, which is the most vital part of this practice.

It is a secret practice that may be uniquely tuned or adjusted by each master to enhance and increase its effectiveness and draw in more energy.

This process is done in a quiet, relaxing space, where the students are asked to close their eyes and focus inside as they receive the attunement.

What happens during the attunement process?

As each attunement progresses in strength from one level to the next, the level of energy that flows into you or that you "tap" into increases in strength as well.

This creates a higher vibration within that causes a variety of effects on each person, which is described in the next section.

Receiving Attunement: What You'll Experience

People describe receiving their first attunement as a spiritual experience, where they are the recipients of a new, positive form of energy.

During and following the process, there are a variety of sensations that the student will experience.

Firstly, it is important to understand how the level of energy flow during each progressive attunement level will increase the level of vibration and power you receive.

This affects each individual differently (or in a similar way), depending on their own unique experience during the process.

The following may be experienced internally during an attunement:

- Colors may appear brighter, and visuals that are clearer and more vibrant than before.

This experience may be temporary or long-term, depending on the individual.

- Some people report seeing angelic beings or similar visuals during an attunement

- Receiving messages and a sense of guidance that is profound and meaningful.

This can give some people a stronger sense of purpose for Reiki and may explain why some practitioners and masters are very passionate about this practice.

- An out-of-body experience or sense of being reborn is one significant experience that may be felt during an attunement.

For some people, this can be a profound, life-changing event where they feel as though they are reborn or starting a new, fresh life.

- A sense of floating or feeling lighter than usual can be another feeling some students experience during the attunement.

In some cases, students report little or no spiritual experience or change, though this doesn't mean that the attunement was unsuccessful.

Every person has varying degrees of energy flow, and while some experiences can be strong and unforgettable, others may be discouraged if they do not feel the same or similar sensations.

Another point of importance to remember is that each attunement session will grow stronger with power, and if one experience doesn't feel as impactful as you expect, this will change from one to the next.

There may also be some ideas or suggestions the Reiki master may be able t to provide to enhance your ability to receive energy during an attunement.

This may include some of the preparations made in-between levels one and two, including cleansing and meditation.

Always remember that attunement is different for everyone, and there is no specific experience, visuals or sensations you need to have for the process to be successful.

Chapter 16: Symbols In Reiki

Symbols are pictorial triggers that are commonly used in meditation as a point of focus or as a tool for visualization in order to achieve a higher sense of awareness and energy manifestation. A symbol aims at the psyche and the subconscious mind to condense the meaning of a whole philosophy into a single symbol.

This same principle is used in Reiki to aid meditation, healing and evoking positive Reiki energy. But it is important to remember that the symbol in itself is not a source of power but the healing treatment and Reiki energy comes from the healer.

Reiki symbols are generally kept secret till the initiate reaches the second level. The symbols for Reiki are based loosely on the Japanese system of writing, Kanji. They are generally taught during the Reiki level 2 - Attunement. However each person is unique and the subconscious of each attunes to these symbols in a different manner based to various factors like intent and psychic energies so it may happen that you may come across variations of these symbols with different Masters. There is no fixed rule for drawing these and therefore nobody is actually wrong.

There are many misunderstandings concerning these symbols, one of which is that they are supposed to draw the symbols in a particular order. These symbols are generally derived from Japanese writing where the style of writing the characters is different from the western world and the writing is done with emphasis on style, direction and order but this is only done for legibility purposes and bears no relevance to the meaning of the symbol or its power in Reiki. Though the Reiki symbols are each used for a specific purpose there are some who prefer to use these symbols combined during Reiki treatments in order to boost the power of the Reiki. This is generally done to make a Reiki healing more effective.

HOW TO MAKE REIKI POWER SYMBOLS WORK FOR YOU!

A reiki course is quite simple in principle: via a simple course of treatment, a student is initiated into the use of reiki energies via a series of ever more precise and powerful 'attunements', which contain a fantastically powerful form manipulating reiki energies effectively. These attunements also have a massively powerful effect on the body, containing and aligning the forces and energies that course through it.

The differing rates at which these energies spin necessitates the partition of reiki courses into three separate levels, according the normal reiki teaching method. In the final stage of reiki instruction, the stage at which the student of reiki finally achieves mastery and the right to use these energies for their personal good and for the good of others, certain reiki power symbols are taught to them by their master. These will be discussed below.

Nowadays, it has become possible, thanks to the Internet and to the explosion of reiki courses throughout the world, to attain the first two levels of reiki mastery within a matter of days. This leads to a stronger reiki attunement, in the experience of respected reiki practitioners. The final control over reiki is signified and carried out by use of the reiki power symbol, which we shall discuss below.

The reiki master attunes the student by acting as a conduit, using his or her hands to alter the energy flows of the student, thereby creating a conduit which allows the energy to flow through the both of them unimpeded.

The cosmic energy that reiki practitioners use is thereby given free play in the body, and the flows from the base of the spine to the top of their head. This river of pure energy is the secret behind the efficacy of reiki energy and the popularity of reiki as a healing method - frequently, both reiki practitioners and patients feel refreshed after a session. This makes these attunements a special experience for both parties, another benefit of reiki.

Stage one of the attunement process, which is meant to benefit the physical, corporeal self of the student, is not where reiki symbols are taught. That comes later, during the second stage, wherein the student is taught the uses of these power symbols as well as the importance of using the right ones for their ends and needs. This attunement opens up the body and allows it access to the spiritual energy contained in the body of the master. The second stage, attunement level 2, is where the reiki symbols are introduced, along with the basic reiki symbol, the reiki power symbol.

Whereas the first stage is intended for the opening up of the energies of the body, the second stage sets the body's energies into motion and gives the student the power to contain them and use them beneficially. So the use of the reiki power symbol lies in stage 2, alongside the distance symbol, and the mental symbol. The power symbol is the basic symbol of the reiki method, as it is what signifies the power of the student over the energies that course through his or her body.

Chapter 17: Who Can Practice Reiki

Reiki is easily learned and practiced as self-care by anyone who is interested, regardless of the person's age or state of health. Children can learn to practice, as can the elderly and the infirm. No special background or credentials are needed to receive training.

One of the hallmarks of Reiki practice is its simplicity, it can be learned in about ten hours of in-person training, generally offered in group class formats, and doesn't require knowledge of either subtle bioenergy or healthcare. It is a wonderful experience to receive Reiki from someone else, a friend or a professional, there are many reasons to consider learning to practice Reiki on yourself.

The convenience of self-care is valued not only by people with health challenges, but also by others with busy schedules who are seeking more balance in their lives.

Additionally, moments of Reiki practice throughout the day can bring centering and relief from pain, anxiety, and stress as often as needed.

People suffering from anxiety or pain who learn Reiki self-care have the additional empowerment of knowing they are never again alone and helpless with their suffering.

Connections To Chakras

Although Reiki and the chakras come from different spiritual and cultural traditions, they have many things in common. Today, many Reiki practitioners use the 7 chakras as an essential part of Reiki healing.

Although some people find this confusing at first, Reiki and the chakra system have more in common than many people realize.

How does Reiki relates to the chakras?

Reiki and the Chakras

Although Reiki and the chakras come from different spiritual and cultural traditions, they have many things in common. Today, many Reiki practitioners use the 7 chakras as an essential part of Reiki healing. Although some people find this confusing at first, Reiki and the chakra system have more in common than many people realize.

What Is Reiki and How Does it Relate to the Chakras?

Reiki is a form of energy healing that originated in Japan. It was discovered by a Buddhist monk named Mikao Usui, who learned to feel and channel the universal life energy that flows through every being. Every person can learn to use this energy for healing by going through a Reiki initiation in which a master awakens the student to Reiki energy.

Since Reiki was first discovered, it has always used the concenpt of energy centers that allow life energy, known as Ki, to move through the body. In the original Japanese tradition, these points are called tandens. Reiki practice originally focused primarily on one energy center, the Seika tanden, which is located in the lower abdomen below the navel. However, there are three tandens. The other two are located in the upper chest and in the center of the forehead.

The chakras, on the other hand, come from Hindu tradition but have also played an important part in Buddhism. The word is Sanskrit for "wheel," although it is often interpreted more as a vortex or whirlpool in energy healing and yogic traditions. The major and minor chakras make up part of the energetic system often referred to as the subtle body along with Kundalini energy that, once awakened, flows through them and activates them. In some traditions, Kundalini awakening must be passed from master to student in a process similar to the Reiki initiation. The primary focus in energy healing is on the seven major chakras, which run up the center of the torso and head and are the main focal points for the meridians, or energy lines, that run through the body.

The minor chakras are smaller focal points where meridians cross. The tandens and the chakra system are simply different interpretations of the same thing. Essentially, they are points that regulate energy flow. If they are blocked or unhealthy, energy cannot flow freely and illness and discomfort result.

Many Reiki healers use the chakra system instead of the tandens. The chakras provide a more detailed energetic map of the body, allowing the healer to focus his or her energy where it is most needed. Although the concept of meridians and energy flow are the same in both systems, the fact that there are seven major chakras can make it easier to provide specific Reiki treatment for physical ailments.

Chakra healing can also help focus emotional and spiritual treatment. The seven chakras each align closely with aspects of mental wellbeing. A Reiki practitioner who has studied the chakra system can use emotional symptoms to help determine where a blockage might have occurred and focus energy on that.Using the chakra system can also help someone who is not a Reiki practitioner take a more active role in their own healing. There are many ways to help balance and open the chakras, including:

Meditation

Yoga

Wearing or using chakra healing stones

Eating certain foods or spices associated with the chakra

Aromatherapy

Each chakra has different elements, colors, foods, and asanas associated with it. By incorporating those elements and practices into daily life in conjuction with Reiki treatment, a person can help speed his or her healing process.In addition, many people find the chakra system more intuitive than the tandens. The colors and symbols associated with it can help with visualizing energy flow and give healers something to help sharpen their focus as they work.

How to do Reiki on Yourself and Others

Self Healing or Treatments are very important when it comes to learning Reiki, at any level .In level 1, you are attuned to receive Reiki, and you are thought the fundamental or basics of how to use it for you own healing and that of your friends and Family.

It is important that you first use it on yourself, for your own self healing and development . Reiki is pure love , it is an act of love to give yourself a Reiki treatment everyday. How many of us, could to do with this in our lives, by giving ourselves 15-30 minutes healing everyday, we give ourselves priority .

By treating on a daily or regular routine, you are keeping the flow of energy flowing through body, which is helping your own healing, by aiding your natural immune system, releasing blocks, this also helps you to understand your own body and helps to improve your intuition, Physically , Energetically , Emotionally and Spiritually you will feel a lot better.

Taking Responsibility: When we give ourselves Self Healing Treatments, we are also taking responsibility for our own healing on every level, even though Reiki can not cure everything, it helps to promote and prioritize our own healing and needs, it does this by teaching us to love our selves unconditionally, it helps us to make changes in our lives, that benefit our health and Well-being . You have often heard the saying " in order to make way for the new, some or all of the old behaviour patterns have to be removed" , and this is what it does , he helps you to realise what's not serving you, and helps you to release it. It trains you , to start looking after yourself, by respecting every aspect of your health and Well-being, helping you to be Happier, Healthier, Physically , Emotionally and Spiritually. When we do this, we are in a much better place, to attract what ever we want in our lives, and this includes helping and treating others, and by showing others how to do the same. This is one of the main Reasons why Doctor Usui started training other people to do Reiki, he found that in early days, the same people kept coming back to him for the same treatments, and they weren't taking responsibly for their own health, so he decided to train some of his clients in Reiki, so they could take responsibility for their health, by using self treatments.

Administering Reiki on yourself: Here for the purposes of First Degree , Level 1 Reiki will show you how to do two Self

Treatments, The Heart and Solar Plexus , which some refer to as the Generic Hand Position for Self Treatment, and a Full Self Treatment.

The Heart and Solar Plexus: In this position you place your Left Hand on Your Heart Chakra and Right Hand on your Solar Plexus, you then Ask and Intend for the Reiki to flow to you , for your highest and greatest, and Say Reiki 3 times, Listen to some music, Sit in Peace, Listen to or Say Affirmations for 15 minutes. Its very easy because you can do it at work, on the bus, When you get up in the morning, or just before you go to sleep at night. Its a very Comforting and Reassuring Treatment, and it also connects you to your Hearts Desire.

Clearing and shielding: This is something you can do on a daily basis, especially if you have been around people a lot, or around harsh situations, or Negative people. The First and Easiest Method, is Sit Quietly and Meditate for a Few, minutes ,

Just to Clear your mind of any internal Chatter, When you have achieved this, take a few deep breaths, and wait, you can feel the Negative or Harsh Energies leaving your with different Sensations, Tingling, or Shivers, or tiny aches and Pains, and your mood gets better and you feel more energised.

Performing reiki on others

You can start healing other people right after being attuned to Reiki degree 1.

As a Reiki 1 channel, you will have to be near the patient you are healing.

After Reiki 2, apart from hands-on healing, you can send anyone Reiki, no matter which part of the world they are.

Hands on Healing: When you are giving hands-on healing to someone, you can either ask them to sit, or lie down. Making them lie down is the most convenient, both for the healer and the patient, as the healer gets comfortable access to all chakras and the patient can relax completely. If the patient communicates with you in advance, ask them to wear comfortable loose-fitting clothes. Once they come for the healing, ask them to remove their spectacles, watch, jewelry, belt, etc. Gold and silver jewelry may be worn. Make sure you and the patient both drink a glass of water. Ask them to lie down comfortably on their back and close their eyes. Start by healing the crown/brow chakra, and then continue to heal all the front chakras.

Once done, balance the energy by spiralling. That is, keep your left hand on their right shoulder, and with your right hand (Index and middle finger extended, thumb touching the ring and little finger) draw anticlockwise spirals starting from the left shoulder, to the tip of the left hand. Next, draw the spirals from the left shoulder to the left foot, then from the right shoulder to the right foot, and then, right shoulder to the tip of right hand.

Ask the patient to turn over the right side and lie on their stomach. Heal the back chakras.

The next step is balancing. Hold your hands above the back brow and back root chakras, about 6 inches above the body. Try to feel the imbalance of energies, and give Reiki till the energy levels feel the same.

Then move your hands slowly to the back throat and back hara chakras. Reiki. Once these chakras are also balanced, move slowly to the back heart and back solar chakras. When these two chakras are balanced, bring both your hands over the back heart chakra and rest it over the body. Keep your left hand on the patient's left shoulder. With the index and middle finger of your right hand, form a V shape and draw a line from the throat to root chakra.

If the patient is diabetic, then draw a line from the root to the throat chakra. Rest your right hand on his/ her back hara chakra. Do this thrice. Gently awaken the patient.

Distance Healing: Distant healing can be done by channels who are attuned to Reiki 2 or above. When you are giving distant healing to someone, it is better to ask them to set some time apart to receive the energy you send them. This increases their energy absorption and will to heal themselves. Ask them to sit with their eyes closed, bare feet touching the floor and without crossing their hands or legs. Let them try to feel the energy coming to them.

There are several ways of sending distant energy. You could use an object as a surrogate, a photograph, an intention slip, imagine them, or send them reiki through your third eye. Each of these points is covered in detail.

Distance Healing Techniques

Using a Photograph: You could ask the patient for a photograph and send reiki energy to the same. Draw the symbols at the back of the photograph and if there is enough space, you might even write above it that their problem is solved. Hold the photograph between your palms and imagine the symbols on it while giving Reiki.

Using a Surrogate: You could use a stuffed toy or a similar object as a surrogate. Mentally declare the toy to be the patient and start giving it Reiki. You can give Reiki to the affected part or give full body Reiki to it. You could also declare small objects or your thumb as the patient, and hold it between your palms and give reiki.

Imagination: Keep your palms cupped together and imagine the person either inside your palms or in front of you, receiving the energy you send and bathing in it. Imagine them feeling better, and draw the symbols while giving them reiki.

Third Eye: If the person is visible, you can imagine reiki energy coming through your third eye and going to that person. Imagine a beam of Reiki coming out through your third eye, and draw the symbols on them with that beam. You could use this technique when you are looking at their photograph or simply imagining that they are standing in front of you and receiving reiki through your third eye.

Intention Slip: You could have an intention box, something which can fit into your palm and contain rolled up papers. Take a small chit of paper and write your intention on one side. Take care to use only positive words (avoid using 'no', 'not', 'don't', 'won't', 'can't', etc), avoid any full stops (period .) and don't fold the paper. After the intention, end it with 'It is so, Thank you Reiki, Thy will be done'. On the opposite side of the paper, draw all the symbols. Roll it up and put it in the intention box. The advantage of the intention box is that you can give Reiki to a lot of people/ events at the same time. Whenever you wish, hold the box between your palms, mentally draw the symbols on it and give Reiki. You don't have to think of all the intentions individually.

Chapter 18: Massive Synchronicity

A few years down the line I had a foreign language student staying with me. As I wanted to add some things to my website, and I had forgotten how to do what was required, I asked his advice. He was a web design student, so when he said as part of his studies he would redesign it, I took him up on his offer. The only problem with this was he went back home to France without telling me how to get into my website or change things myself. I was not so happy with my site after his changes and determined to learn how to do this myself which was to take time. I decided to do a night class at my local college so that if I got someone to redesign my website, I would then be able to keep it up to date by understanding what I was doing.

At college, I learned that he had changed the operating system of my website, but only some of it. This meant it was more messed up than I had been aware of. The Lecturer was shocked that my website was still working. I knew to get a new website made was going to cost me a lot of money that I did not have. The alternate was one of the cheap ones which looked very unprofessional at that time. I found the course interesting but was then in over my head after a few weeks when the lecturer concentrated on teaching Dreamweaver. At that point he lost me. I was feeling disheartened with my course and wondering what I should do moving forward. Around this time a massive piece of synchronicity happened. I had a call from my son who worked inside a web design company. He advised me that he had someone willing to make me a website for free as he already had a template for a similar one. I was so pleased to feel that soon I would be the happy owner of a professional well-designed website that of course I said yes.

I got a lot more than I thought and ended up with my fantastic website.

The fabulous thing was my website was designed by the person who had created the original template. He was also good at optimising websites so that they could be found. The only cost to me was a reiki treatment for his wife and I added in a pregnancy massage from my friend for her also. The universe was really helping me to move forward. After this I had therapists in other countries contacting me to say what they thought of my website. People who knew me said it was just right for me. This person, for quite a while after, even helped maintain my website while teaching my son how to do the job also. To this day I call upon my son when I need help although he has advised me, I need to check YouTube first for any answers. It's amazing what you can find on that site.

I decided that to go with my super new website I needed special business cards. When I had been out with my dog, I came across a bench in memory of someone and the words resonated with me. Every time I passed, I had to read them as I kept feeling a pull towards them. I later learned they were written by Ralph Waldo Emerson. "Do not go where the path may lead, go instead where there is no path and leave a trail."

I really felt as if I was started on a new journey, a new way of life. I wanted to do it my way and felt that many changes were coming.

Synchronicity Rules!

I owe the way I run my workshops to my teacher. At the time he taught me, he always had very small groups of people in his workshops. This made it a very informal enjoyable way of learning. I am happy to teach someone reiki as an individual or in very small groups - usually no more than eight. I feel it is a joyous thing to learn and the day should be taken at the pace that is right for the individuals. During one period synchronicity played a big part in my reiki workshops.

I received a call for someone wishing to book a reiki session. This person had Myalgic Encephalopathy (M.E.). The next week my friend who also had M.E asked for the same. A couple of weeks later I had someone with M.E asking to use the chi machine. Do you think the universe was trying to tell me something? This is when something happened that blew me away. A local M.E charity contacted me to say they had been given a grant to train people in different types of therapies, so they would be able to help others with this illness. They asked if I would like to train two people. The interesting thing was none of the many people that were going to be trained knew which therapy they were to be trained in.

I advised that reiki was different in that it affects you both mentally and spiritually in many ways and people should be aware of this if they wanted to take part. She did advise that a previous person had decided after level one training not to go on to the next level. I said that I would want to make sure that the people chosen knew how they may be affected as it was not like massage when you could just learn the strokes. (No disrespect to massage therapists intended). With reiki, the mind / spirit is involved also. She then advised me she would be giving the students the contact telephone numbers of four other reiki teachers and would advise them to decide, after speaking to them all, who they wanted to be trained by. A week later I had just come home at lunchtime when the first person called me, and we spoke for a while. A few days later I had just come home for a short while later in the afternoon when the second person called me, and again we spoke for some time. Later I was talking to a friend and I advised I knew the students were going to choose me. When she asked how I knew, I said that there was only one hour out of each of those days at different times when I was at home, and they both called during that time. Sure enough, they each called back with an affirmative to be trained by me. One of them called while I was talking to a group of people about synchronicity and about all my M.E experiences! The next bit of synchronicity was when they met outside my home and found that they both knew each other. What a brilliant start to the day.

We had arranged a training day starting a bit later in the day and allowed their health to dictate the speed of the training. I found I was much more tired than usual at the end of the day as the pace was quite slow. Over the next few days both contacted me to go over little bits as the memories of people that have M.E are often impaired. This is where only teaching small groups comes into its own. It means that I have time for people who need extra help and support.

A few months later they came back for level two training. As this was over a couple of days, I had to completely change how I actioned my training that weekend. At the end of it and after they had done their homework over the next four weeks, I was pleased to have two reiki practitioners now ready to help their charity. The special point of reiki level two was to enable them to send distance reiki when someone with M.E was too ill to receive a visit. One of them called me a couple of weeks later to advise he had just had a massive coincidence. He had gone to a shopping centre and was going around and around in circles looking for a parking space. Out of the corner of his eye he saw a space become available, so he drove in to it. When he got out of his car, he was astounded to see the car next to him had the number plate Joy so told me I must have been watching out for him. He also said when I was writing my story, I had to add his story into it, so this is for you Jeff Begg. Unfortunately, Jeff passed away before I got this book published.

Most of the time I can accept whatever life gives me but if I struggle at any point I can go and meditate for a while and give myself reiki and it all comes back into perspective again. Reiki is a tool that is with me whenever I need it. The thing I am most pleased about though is how relaxed and chilled out I feel. I now have a much more positive attitude to everything, which has enabled me to write articles about this very subject. You can check out some of these at my website: https://peaceharmonyandjoy.co.uk/category/blog/ I'll say it again and again - "I love reiki".

Orbs

One summer I was asked for a photo of me working for a charity newsletter. As I was hosting foreign language students one said he would take some photographs for me, so I went and got my neighbour to come through to my house. We tried posing with the therapy table in different areas of the room trying to get good snaps while having quite a few giggles in the process. At one point I felt the energy kick in and she did also. I remember her telling me I was not meant to be treating her at that time, so we had a laugh. It just shows that the energy can decide when to make an appearance without being invited. The interesting thing is when the photographs were uploaded to my computer there were orbs in the ones at exactly the points where we felt the energy kick in. When I uploaded this photo to Face book it was pointed out that there was also another orb there too.

Orbs are nothing new in my house. I had my last dog Misty until she was almost 12 years of age. During this time, she would often stare into the air as if she could see something I could not. It used to freak out some visitors although regulars would just say "She's at it again!" This was before I really knew about spiritual orbs but on looking back at photographs of her, she was often surrounded by them. I remember two friends dog sitting for me and they took a photograph of Misty. Sure enough, there were orbs around her. They wanted to know if she had brought them to their house. Animals can be very spiritual and intuitive. Misty sure was and is still around me today.

I remember going to a place near Edinburgh called Rosslyn Chapel with other people that I met. A lot of people connect Rosslyn with the Knights Templar. We had all been on David's Facebook page as he had trained us all at different times. Two of them, who I had never met before, invited me the next day to the Chapel. They decided to visit a cave situated below the Chapel and asked if I wished to go there too. That was a day of experiences.

When we went to the road, we found it blocked off with large metal gates. There was a very small space between the edge of the gate and the road. One of them pulled out a space blanket and laid it on the ground under the gate. We then, with a bit of trepidation, all crawled underneath it. On the way to the cave we stopped at a tree. One of the ladies explained it was so twisted due to a vortex. At this point she brought out divining rods and crystal pendulums. It was interesting to see them all at work.When we got to the cave it was so dark that I could not see inside it. One of the ladies gave me a singing bowl. I was astonished to see that while I used it, the cave was brighter, and I could see right to the back of it. As soon as I stopped, it went dark again. Both ladies felt the presence of spirits while they were inside. We had taken a few photographs and found, when they were uploaded to a computer, that there were Orbs exactly at the points they both felt Spirits!

I remember after that we decided to go for a meal at a hotel nearby. I was walking towards it still trying to get the mud off my clothes! That was a day of experiences for me that will forever stay in my memory.

Conclusion

The mystery of the Sahara Yoga method dwells within us, at the base of the spinal harmony, in a triangular bone called the "sacrum bone". Since our introduction to the world in our sacrum bone dwells an inner vitality brought in Sanskrit Kundalini; it is portrayed as a feminine vitality and once initiated, this vitality rises along our spine until it achieves the highest point of the head and finally associates with the all inclusive vitality. This union is called "yoga" in Sanskrit.

When you're under stress, muscles strained and breathing becomes shallow and fast. When you breathe gradually and profoundly, it makes an impression on your brain to quiet down. The brain then sends this message to your body. Profound breathing increases the oxygen accessible to your body and delivers a casual feeling. Rehearse this strategy a couple times every day, and profound breathing will become a tool you can use to offer you some assistance with relaxing at whatever point you feel stressed.

www.ingramcontent.com/pod-product-compliance
Lightning Source LLC
Chambersburg PA
CBHW072011070526
44583CB00015B/1439